How to
Make Love
All Night

Also by Barbara Keesling, Ph.D.

*Sexual Pleasure: Reaching New Heights of
Sexual Arousal and Intimacy*

How to Make Love All Night
(and Drive a Woman Wild)

MALE MULTIPLE ORGASM AND OTHER SECRETS FOR PROLONGED LOVEMAKING

BARBARA KEESLING, Ph.D.

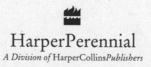

HarperPerennial

A Division of HarperCollinsPublishers

A hardcover edition of this book was published in 1994 by HarperCollins Publishers.

HarperCollins books may be purchased for educational, business, or sales promotional use. For information please write: Special Markets Department, HarperCollins Publishers, Inc., 10 East 53rd Street, New York, NY 10022.

First HarperPerennial edition published 1995.

Designed by Nancy Singer

The Library of Congress has catalogued the hardcover edition as follows:

Keesling, Barbara.
    How to make love all night (and drive a woman wild) : male multiple orgasm and other secrets for prolonged lovemaking / Barbara Keesling. — 1st ed.
        p. cm.
    Includes bibliographical references.
    ISBN 0-06-017122-7
    1. Sex instruction for men. 2. Male orgasm. I. Title.
HQ36.K44 1994
613.9'6'024041—dc20   94-9703

ISBN 0-06-092621-X (pbk.)
 97 98 99 ❖/HC 10 9 8 7

This book is dedicated
to my clients.

Contents

Introduction   ix

Acknowledgments   xi

ONE   Making Fantasy a Reality   1

TWO   Meet Your Penis   17

THREE   Talking to Your Partner About Male
Multiple Orgasm   29

FOUR   The Complete PC Workout   43

FIVE   Male Multiple Orgasm—
The Secret Revealed   51

SIX   Learning to Touch, Learning
to Feel   67

SEVEN   Aroused and Aware   81

EIGHT   Orgasm, Ejaculation, and You   95

NINE   From Peaks to Plateaus   107

TEN   Your First Multiple Orgasm   119

ELEVEN   Practice, Practice, Practice   151

TWELVE   Success!   161

**APPENDIX
ONE**   Interesting Things to Read
When You're Not Having Sex   173

**APPENDIX
TWO**   Male Sexual Organs
(diagram)   177

Introduction

Daniel and Allison have been making love on a rainy Sunday morning, and they are both totally turned on. It started in the shower with a slow massage and moved to the bedroom, where they have been having intercourse for the past ten minutes. Daniel knows that Allison needs at least another five minutes of intercourse before she can climax. Here's the problem: Daniel doesn't think he has five minutes left in him.

If Daniel continues having intercourse the way he has for the past ten minutes, it may be only a matter of seconds before he has an orgasm. He thinks about slowing down or stopping, but to break the rhythm now would only make it more difficult for Allison to climax—he knows that Allison is at that stage where any kind of change in his movement would only frustrate her. Besides, if he tried to stop or to change the rhythm, Daniel could lose strength in his erection, which would complicate matters even further.

This dilemma is making the whole experience a lot less pleasurable for Daniel. The first few minutes of sex were pure excitement, but now he is worried and conflicted. It is hard to enjoy sex when you're fighting your own body. Truth is, you really *can't* enjoy sex when you're fighting your own body. And neither can your partner.

What Daniel does not yet know is that he has another option: *male multiple orgasm*. The multiorgasmic man has staying power. He doesn't have to hold back. He doesn't have to fight his own body and deny himself his own pleasure. He can enjoy all of the erotic sensations of intercourse, have a full orgasm, *and keep going!* If he wishes, he can have a second orgasm, *and keep going!* He can last as long as his partner wishes, experience all of the excitement and release, *and keep going!* For the multiorgasmic man, the sky is truly the limit.

Daniel is not the only man who has this exciting option. Today, techniques have been perfected to make male multiple orgasm an option for almost *every man!* Age doesn't matter. Previous experience doesn't matter. Young or old, virgin or veteran, all you need is the desire, your penis, and a few minutes a day. So don't stop now. Turn the page and cross the threshold into a whole new sense of your own sexuality and a whole new relationship for you and your partner.

Acknowledgments

There are many people I would like to thank.

First, I wish to thank my colleagues, Anita Banker and Michael Riskin, for helping develop many of these techniques.

I would like to thank my agent, Barbara Lowenstein, for recognizing the value of this project.

I wish to thank my editor, Susan Moldow, and her staff, Nancy Peske and Wendy Silbert, for their very conscientious work on this book.

I would especially like to thank my clients who tried out these techniques and gave me their invaluable feedback

Finally, I would like to thank my husband, John, for his computer work, his feedback on the manuscript, and his support.

Some of the exercises in this book involve orgasm. Having an orgasm increases your heart rate. If you have a heart condition or any other serious medical condition, please consult your physician before beginning this or any other exercise program.

CHAPTER ONE

Making Fantasy a Reality

Every woman dreams of being with a lover whose passion is so intense and body is so strong that he can last and last and last. Every man wants to be able to fulfill those dreams. He wants to know that he can have intercourse for as long as he wishes, bringing his partner to climax after climax. It certainly sounds wonderful, but is it possible?

You are about to learn the secrets of male multiple orgasm. By the time you have completed this book, your understanding of sexual potential and sexual power will be changed forever. You will learn how to prolong lovemaking for as long as you and your partner desire. Men will learn how to master their own bodies. They will learn how to have complete, powerful orgasms without losing their erections, and how to have multiple orgasms—two, three, or even more—just like a woman.

I know that this may be hard to believe. It's hard to imagine that such sexual powers could exist for *anyone*. Maybe for a twenty-year-old with unlimited energy or some yogi with extraordinary abilities, or maybe at the beginning of a torrid love affair, if you should be so lucky. But not for your average guy. No, for most normal men with normal sexual equipment, it seems like making love all night whenever you want—no matter how long you've been married or how old you are—is a fantasy. Until today. Today, everything is going to change; today, those fantasies are going to come true.

In this book, I'm going to teach men how to explore and enjoy their sexuality in ways they may not have believed possible. I'm going to prove to you that male multiple orgasm is not just part of some romance writer's imagination, but an easily attainable reality. You are going to discover how a multiorgasmic man can offer his partner a level of pleasure and fulfillment more intense than either one of them could have ever hoped for.

The ability to control one's penis—to literally stay up all night—is not the exclusive domain of Eastern masters. There are plenty of men who have already learned to control their erections in ways you would find hard to imagine. These men can have multiple orgasms without losing their erections (two orgasms, three orgasms, or even more if they choose). They drive their women wild hour after hour, night after night. They're doing it right now—and they'll still be doing it long after you've gone to sleep.

These men are not sexual supermen. They are normal, average guys. Some are young, some are old, some are tall, some are small, some are thin, some are overweight, some are bashful, and some are bold. Some have large penises, some have small penises, some have thick penises, and some have slender penises. Some have sex once a week, and some have sex almost every day. The only thing these men all have in common is the desire to please themselves and pleasure their partners, and the discipline to master a simple technique.

I know over two hundred of these men personally. They are not friends or lovers, but they are men who have learned the secrets of male multiple orgasm and staying power at the various therapy clinics where I have worked. Over the past ten years, I have had the opportunity to train more than one hundred of these men, one on one, from start to finish. The rest are men whose training and progress I have been at least partially involved with through my clinical work.

What I'm trying to say, without sounding intimidating or otherwise off-putting, is that I have seen many men become multiorgasmic and increase their staying power. And there is something extremely important you need to know before you read any further: *I have never met a motivated man who couldn't master the techniques that lead to male multiple orgasm. Never.* I *know* that every man who reads this book and follows the exercises I describe can master these techniques too.

If you are a woman reading this book, extraordinary surprises and unimaginable pleasures await you. Whether you choose to work with your partner as he learns these techniques, or be a supportive bystander, your understanding of what it means to be intimate with a man is about to be redefined forever.

If you are a man reading this book, you are about to enter into a new relationship—a new and exciting relationship with your own penis. You will never be the same. The payoffs are unlimited—payoffs for you, payoffs for your partner, and payoffs for your relationship. By the time you finish this book and complete the simple exercises I describe, you *will* be a changed man. After you've had your first multiple orgasm, you won't believe you waited this long, but you will believe in yourself and in the power of your own sexuality.

What Makes Me Such an Expert?

I know more about men's penises than most men do. It's my job. I'm a sex therapist.

I'm also a former sex surrogate. A female sex surrogate is someone who teaches men how to control and improve their sexual performance and enjoy their own sexuality.

To be a sex surrogate you have to know men and you have to know men's penises. Truth is, you have to know men's penises better than most men do. Sure, the typical man knows what he likes and dislikes, he knows his strengths and weaknesses, and he may even be keenly aware of his fears and what he believes to be his limitations. But from where I sit, this awareness is very limited. When you work with hundreds of men, you see things that no one man could ever see for himself. You recognize how easy it is for a man to have sexual tunnel vision because of the limitations of his own experience. You also realize how different men are, and how much there is to learn from the experiences of other men.

I Know What Men Can Do and I Know What Women Want

I have made the study of human sexual response my life's work. I know what the average man's *true* capabilities are, and believe me, they are far more than you could ever imagine.

I know what women want too because I'm not just a sex therapist—I'm also a woman. I understand how a woman feels when she's in bed with someone she loves. On a professional basis, I've listened to countless women talk about their lovemaking. But even more revealing in some ways are the hours I have spent talking about sex with women friends, all of us letting our hair down and telling the truth about what we like and what we want.

Even a woman who loves a man very deeply can feel frustrated and unfulfilled by his sexual limitations. Unfortunately, many women equate sex with compromise and sacrifice. Few women regularly experience the kind of lovemaking they dream of, and even fewer believe it's actually possible. That's the bad news. The good news is that this is about to change.

If you are a woman looking for more satisfaction from your partner and more understanding for yourself, I'm going to teach you everything you and your partner need to know about male multiple orgasm. If you are a man who is reading this book, I want you to think of me as a personal trainer—someone who can teach you the techniques and exercises that will change everything you have ever believed about sex.

Can We Talk?

Remember that big "talk" you had about sex with your dad when you were just a kid? Who could forget it? It was probably one of the most awkward moments of your childhood, right? Sure he did the best he could, but you probably were left to fill in a whole lot of gaps by yourself. Well, it's time for another talk. This time, *you* and *I* need to talk about sex . . . really talk. If you have a partner, she should listen too. I'm not going to pull any punches here. When it comes to sex, there are a lot of things most people just don't know. I'm not talking about sexual trivia—I'm talking about the critical things that stop most people from ever having a truly fulfilling sex life.

Please don't get insulted. I know that you know a lot about sex. Everyone does, whether they want to or not. After all, it's a subject that's hard to avoid in the nineties. Turn on the TV, plug in the radio, open a book, go to the movies, flip through a magazine . . . what do you see? Sex, sex, sex. From Howard Stern to Melrose Place, from Donahue to pay-per-view, we're getting educated by osmosis. But that doesn't mean it's a very *good* education.

Knowing a lot about sex is not the same as being sexually fulfilled. Knowing a lot about sex doesn't always change what happens in the bedroom. No matter how much you've heard, read, and seen, sex can still feel like the greatest mystery in the world. No one likes to feel insecure about something as important as sex, but the truth is, at some point everyone feels as though everyone else on the planet is making love more often and more exquisitely than they are. Sometimes it feels as though all of this sexual education has only made us more unsure.

It's time to change all that and start filling in all of those gaps once and for all. I couldn't think of a better place to start than learning about male multiple orgasm, which will change everything you ever thought you knew about sex. In fact, it will change everything. Period. It certainly did for me and for the many men and women with whom I've worked. I'm sure it will for you too.

Two Men Who Changed My
Understanding of Male Sexuality

Male multiple orgasm. Wow! What a concept. I'll
never forget how skeptical I felt when I first heard
about it back in 1980. It was my second week of
"basic training" for sexual surrogates at the Riskin-
Banker Psychotherapy Center in Tustin, California.

Sex therapy is an important area of specializa-
tion at Riskin-Banker, and part of their therapeutic
work involves the use of surrogates, both male and
female. As it turns out, two of the male surrogates
who worked there at the time were both capable of
achieving multiple orgasm. On certain occasions,
they actually used these techniques during work
with their female clients.

If I hadn't actually known these two men personally, I might have never believed such a thing
was possible. Sure, I knew all about multiple
orgasm in women. But men? How could men have
multiple orgasms? I had a million questions that
needed answering. As I listened to each of these
men talk in detail about their unusual abilities, I
knew that my understanding of male sexuality was
about to change radically and permanently.

By the time my training was complete, I had all
the proof of male multiple orgasm I ever needed.
Since then I have spent most of my time working
hard with other clinicians and clients to develop and
perfect a variety of techniques that any man or couple could practice in the comfort of their own home.
Today, I want to share those techniques with you.
Why? Because I care about relationships and I care
about sex. We need to have good sex in our relation-

ships. Good sex brings us closer together. It strengthens intimacy and cements the bond. It can even save a marriage. We can't try to hide from this. Quite the contrary—we need to do everything we can to celebrate the importance of a rich sexual connection.

Are You Ready for a Change Too?

Is the possibility of a truly exciting sex life the kind of news you've been waiting for, or does it all sound too good to be true? For some people, the concept of male multiple orgasm seems perfectly logical, but to others, it may seem somewhat unnatural, or even downright impossible.

If you're feeling a bit skeptical or uneasy right now, that's normal. It has to be somewhat disconcerting to think we don't know such a vital piece of sexual information. But as any good sex therapist will confirm for you, new sexual techniques are being developed all the time as we discover more about our bodies and our sexual capabilities. These new discoveries can be intimidating at first, but ultimately they're very good news for all of us.

So relax if you can and try to be as open as possible. Believe me, even if you have your doubts right now, they won't last. I'm not here to teach you theory, but to deliver the goods. By the time you have finished the exercises in this book, I know you will be a believer, with all the proof you ever need right in your own hands. Literally.

Was That a Smile I Just Saw?

I hope that by now I've already made you smile, or even laugh. We all need to laugh a little bit more about sex, and I believe in using humor to help people learn about sex. Don't get me wrong—I'm not a comedienne. I have a Ph.D. in psychology and I take sex very seriously—so you don't have to.

I like sex and I believe in sex. I think it's one of the most wonderful things that can happen between a man and a woman. I think its value to a relationship is immeasurable. But I also think we need to be able to laugh about sex and during sex. Here's my bottom line: I believe that sex should be easy and wonderful and fun for everyone. Having sex should be like going to Disneyland—tons of different rides, plenty to eat, and fireworks at midnight—only better because you don't have to wait on line. Does that sound good to you?

Why Are You Reading This Book?

If you are a woman reading this book, you probably have several reasons for doing so. Because you love your partner a lot, you care about giving him as much pleasure as possible in bed. You want him to be the best lover he can be, but not just so he can fulfill your physical needs. You want him to feel good about himself in all ways; you want to be able to tell him that he's a fabulous lover, and have him know for himself that it's true.

But you also probably have some selfish reasons for being interested in male multiple orgasm. Perhaps you're feeling frustrated because most, if not all, of your orgasms are reached through oral sex or clitoral stimulation without penetration. Perhaps you want to be able to know that your partner can sustain an erection long enough to give you the stimulation you need to achieve orgasm through intercourse. Or perhaps, even if you're satisfied with the quality of your orgasms, you want to be able to spend more time making love. Maybe you simply find so much joy in having sex with your partner that you want to be able to do it longer. There is nothing wrong with wanting to make your sex life more and more wonderful. Too many women settle for less than what they really want, and I'm glad you're not one of them.

If you are a man reading this book, I know that you care about making your partner happy in bed and are sensitive to a woman's sexual needs. You want her to feel fulfilled and satisfied, and that's terrific. If you didn't, you wouldn't be interested in what I have to say. Perhaps you are already able to make love for an extended period of time, and you're reading this because you want to intensify your pleasure or want to find other ways of expressing your sexuality. Perhaps you are anxious about your ability to maintain an erection, or you would like to experience a greater intensity in your own sexual response. Perhaps you are trying to rediscover the multiorgasmic ability that you had as a younger man, or re-create an isolated multiorgasmic experience in your past that left you wanting more. Perhaps you are just curious.

Whatever your reasons, you are about to discover the wonderful things that becoming multiorgasmic does for a man. It's not just your body that will be changing. Your sense of who you are is going to change, and so is your sense of what you have to offer a woman. When a man feels good about his sexuality, he feels good about himself. Sexual confidence creates greater confidence in many other areas of a man's life. It strengthens self-image and it strengthens self-esteem. This is powerful stuff.

Four Typical Men Who Want to Learn About Male Multiple Orgasm

You've already met Daniel. Right now, I'd like to introduce you to four other men: Fred, David, Josh, and Mark. As you will see, each of these men has a different reason for wanting to learn about male multiple orgasm, and every reason is valid. Maybe you will recognize some of your own needs and concerns in one of their stories. I think *most* men have something in common with at least one of these four men.

FRED'S STORY

Fred has always found it very easy to express his sexuality. He is currently married for the second time and he and his wife Janice have a very active sex life. Because sex is important to Fred, he wants to make sure it stays that way.

Right now, he and Janice make love almost every night and many mornings as well. Fred says that to him it's sort of like brushing his teeth—something you do routinely at regular intervals of the day. But Fred is becoming worried that his "refractory period"—the length of time between erections—is getting longer. Or, as Fred puts it, "Lately, I can't always get it up twice a day." Fred is interested in finding new techniques that will allow him to continue to spend large amounts of time having sex with his wife. Janice thinks that's a pretty good idea.

DAVID'S STORY

David has a completely different reason for being interested in learning about male multiple orgasm. He worries that he can't keep an erection long enough to satisfy his wife, Debbie, and he's concerned that she is not as happy in bed as she would like to be. It seems that no matter how hard David tries, he can't sustain an erection for much longer than five minutes. He laughs when he refers to himself as "a quickie," but he doesn't really think it's funny. He's willing to try anything that will bring Debbie to orgasm, but he knows what his wife really needs is prolonged intercourse.

In truth, David never had much control over his erection, but when he and Debbie first started sleeping together he felt so much desire that after he reached orgasm he was able to have a second erection within ten or fifteen minutes. The second time, it was easier for him to hold back his own orgasm and ejaculation, allowing him to prolong intercourse long enough for Debbie to reach orgasm. Over time, however, David lost this ability, and that's been a problem for Debbie.

Debbie agrees. David has read several books that promise he can become a great lover by learning to press the right spots on a woman's body. But when he tries these techniques on Debbie, they don't really seem to be working. They don't work because other books don't explain the philosophy behind the techniques, and David ends up "working on" Debbie instead of enjoying himself.

Touching is nice, and oral sex is great, but Debbie needs more intercourse to feel satisfied. She misses the long sessions of lovemaking. Sometimes she feels that she is just beginning to get excited as David is already ejaculating. Knowing that this is going to happen makes her nervous and uncomfortable when they're having intercourse. She feels as though she is spending more time thinking about David's erection than she is about her own pleasure. She loves David and she doesn't want to hurt his feelings, so she gasps and moans and pretends to have an orgasm. But it's not the same, and she knows it. Worse still, he knows it.

Both Debbie and David want the same thing: sex that is passionate and prolonged. They want to feel comfortable with themselves and with each other. David wants desperately to last long enough to bring his wife to orgasm through intercourse. When he thinks of making love to her, in his head he can continue for hours. Why doesn't that happen in real life? By using the technique of male multiple orgasm, it can.

Josh and Mark

Mark has yet another set of reasons for wanting to learn about male multiple orgasm. Still a young man, Mark has yet to find a steady partner, and he has anxiety about his ability to perform well when he does. He wants to learn as much about sex as he can so that he will feel more secure and knowledgeable when he is with women.

Josh is only a few years older than Mark, but he considers himself very experienced sexually. He thinks of himself as a good lover and believes that he is able to maintain an erection long enough to satisfy any partner. But Josh has another concern: he is so mentally aware of "holding back" his orgasms in order to please the woman he's with that it keeps him from fully enjoying the experience.

Until very recently, all of these men believed there was only one secret involved in being a good lover: "learning to play a woman's body like a violin." But that has all changed now. Today, these four men are enthusiastic and excited, having discovered that there is yet another secret that will allow them to bring pleasure to their partners while increasing their own pleasure.

What about you? Aren't you tired of those violin lessons too? And if you're a woman, aren't you tired of being treated like a string instrument? Are you ready to finally learn something that can really make a difference in your sex life? I think you are. I think you've been ready for a long, long time.

So where do we begin? It is my experience that before a man can learn to have his first multiple orgasm he needs to learn a little bit more about himself. More specifically, he needs to develop a new, more sophisticated understanding of the main character in this book: his penis. With that in mind, it's time to turn the page and take a new look at a very old friend. . . .

CHAPTER TWO

Meet Your Penis

efore we go any further, I need to talk to you about your penis. Traditionally, men are intensely preoccupied with trying to learn the secret of mastering women's bodies, yet they spend so little time trying to understand their own. The typical man is prepared to burn the midnight oil studying the intricacies of the female anatomy. He will happily pick up a flashlight and search endlessly for G spots, sun spots, or any other spots that will help him be a better lover, yet he barely knows his own equipment. There's only one thing wrong with that: you can't become multiorgasmic if you don't know your own penis.

A Penis Is a Terrible Thing to Waste

Do you like your penis? Are you proud of it? Or are your positive feelings mixed with feelings of embarrassment, shame, and doubt? Don't feel bad if they are. The truth is, it's a rare man who is truly comfortable with his own penis. When it comes to their most private parts, most men feel extremely self-conscious and extremely vulnerable.

We need to change that. Why? Because a positive attitude about your own body is going to set the stage for a radical change in your sexual power. Every man needs to understand the following fact: the secret to being a good lover lies not within a woman's body, but within his own. *Any man can become a phenomenal lover if he understands that his greatest sexual power lies in his ability to understand and control his own penis.*

If you want to become a sexual virtuoso, the first thing you need to do is master your own penis. Everything else will follow very quickly from there. To ignore the power of your own penis is to waste your greatest asset, and that's a shame.

Aren't You Tired of Having Sex with a Stranger?

You have known your penis all your life. You have known your penis longer than you have known your partner, your boss, your best friend, or your trusty dog Spuds. Yet, for all the time you've been together, you barely know it at all. Even though you probably take a good look at your equipment every single day, the real potential of your own penis has continued to elude you.

When was the last time you spent any quality time with your penis? When was the last time you two had a real heart-to-heart? I'd guess you were probably eleven or twelve years old at the time. Chances are that back then you were fascinated with your own equipment. It didn't seem like there was enough time in the day for the two of you to get to know one another. But once you had your first few orgasms, that probably started to change. Once you discovered what felt good to you at the time, your curiosity began to wane. You found a formula that worked, you stuck with it, and that was that.

Even if you were tempted to experiment over the years, your attempts were probably more frustrating than fulfilling. A lack of helpful information and an abundance of misinformation could only discourage your natural interest. Living in a world with so little to offer you, you did the best you could. You made peace with your penis and forged a working relationship that continues to this day. Sure, you might have tried something new once in a great while when you met a new partner or when you got a little bored, but chances are that ten, twenty-five, or even fifty years later, you're doing pretty much the same thing that you did as an eleven-year-old.

But you're not eleven anymore. You've grown up and your body has grown up. Your needs have changed, and now you have a partner who also has needs. Don't you think it's time to develop an adult understanding of your own equipment? Don't you think it's time to expand upon the mindset of that enthusiastic but naive eleven-year-old and get excited again about your sexual potential as a man?

Does Your Penis Have a Mind of Its Own?

In this chapter, I'm going to help you take the first step toward becoming more intimate with your penis. You are going to realize, probably for the first time, how you can gain control of your own equipment. This is a big switch for any man who believes it is his penis that is always at the helm.

Men typically treat their penises as though they were separate, disconnected objects with brains of their own. They say things like, "Don't talk to me

. . . talk to *him*. *He* did it." They give their penises names like "Little Robert," "Big Jim," "Captain Fantastic," or "Mr. Doozy." I have to admit, this really makes me laugh because women are so different. How many women do you know who have pet names for their vaginas? How many times do you hear women affectionately refer to their genitals using names like "Miss Lucy" or "The Cannibal"? You don't hear women saying things like, "I guess little Beth down there doesn't want to come out to play today."

There are lots of possible reasons why men treat their penises in this disconnected fashion. No doubt, there are some men who split themselves off from their penises because they don't want to take responsibility for their own sexuality or the consequences of their own sexual behavior. It's a great way to justify being careless or insensitive. I think even more men distance themselves from their genitals because they have problems dealing with the frustration of being unable to control their bodies. This makes any perceived sexual failures or perceived shortcomings easier to tolerate.

Because the penis is physically externalized—hanging out there, so to speak—it is more open to scrutiny. If a woman fails to get aroused, only she knows for sure. She may not be happy about it, but you won't read about it in the tabloids. Not so for a man. If a penis isn't doing what it's supposed to do, everyone in the room knows it. If a man is having difficulties, the evidence is out there in the open for all to see. Even those satellites in outer space that photograph license plates are going to recognize a

penis that isn't doing its job. That's a lot of pressure—too much pressure for the average man.

Your New Best Friend

It may be easier to think your penis has its own personality, but a disconnected attitude like this ultimately will not serve you well. It may spare you
some anxiety and discomfort, but it also robs you of
much of your pleasure.

Your penis is not a separate entity subletting
space in your underwear. It is not that noisy tenant
downstairs who keeps you awake all night long.
Don't treat it that way. Your penis is an important
part of you; it's sometimes the most honest part of
you. When you're scared, your penis shows it. When
you're excited, your penis shows it. When you're
depressed, your penis knows it, and it behaves
accordingly. You can fool some of the people some
of the time, but you can't fool your own penis. The
two of you are totally connected, and you will be for
the rest of your life. Now that's no stranger, is it?

I tell men: Embrace your penis! Put out the welcome mat. Open a dialogue. Let it know it's a part
of you and let it know you care. It's time to bring
your penis in from the cold. The sooner you do, the
sooner your sexuality will start to change. Now
here's the best news. If you like your penis, your
partner is going to like your penis. If you're proud
of your penis, your partner is going to be proud of
your penis. If you embrace your penis, your partner
is going to embrace your penis. Sound good? I
thought it would.

A Man Who Controls His Penis Is a Man in Demand

In my experience, there are two kinds of men in the world: men who control their penises and men who are controlled by their penises. A man who cannot control his penis is a man who lives in fear. He fears having his inadequacy discovered, not being able to have a satisfying sex life, and not being able to fulfill the woman he loves.

For all of us—male and female—the single greatest obstacle to sexual pleasure is fear of our own equipment. My goal is to begin dismantling some of that fear. A healthier relationship with one's penis can dissolve many common performance anxieties by giving a man a true sense of control over his own functioning.

Sexual performance is not a mystery or something to be feared. Sexual functioning is a physiological process, just like breathing or sleeping—it just feels better. Like most other physiological processes, your sexual performance can be understood, altered, and improved. And that's exactly what you are going to do, starting today.

An Important Anatomy Lesson

Everybody knows that the penis is not a muscle. If it was, you'd probably be at the gym right now. What most people don't know is that there *is* a muscle that plays a crucial role in the functioning of the penis: the pubococcygeus muscle (pyoo-bo-cock-see-gee-us). Say that five times fast.

The pubococcygeus muscle—or PC muscle, for short—is actually a group of muscles that run from the pubic bone to the tailbone. Now, you may already know this muscle in a different way. The PC muscle is the muscle you use to stop the flow of urine from the bladder. It is also the muscle that contracts when you ejaculate, moving the semen up through the penis and out of the body.

The PC muscle is a busy little muscle. But let me tell you, as far as most men are concerned, it is still grossly underemployed. Don't you worry—we're going to change all that very soon. *Male multiple orgasm depends on a strong PC muscle.* The PC muscle is the key to penile reformation. It's your ticket to the big leagues . . . your way to the top. Most of the techniques you will learn in later chapters cannot be done without PC power. That's why the first set of exercises I introduce in this book is designed specifically to "prep" the PC muscle. *These exercises, found in chapter 4, are crucial and must be done first.* They cannot be skipped and they cannot be taken lightly. So don't skip them, and don't take them lightly. Please.

Power to the PC

Now you may be thinking, "I'm not eighteen any-more. My penis doesn't function like the penis of a younger man, exercise or no exercise." Listen to me. It doesn't matter how old or young you are. Is an eighteen-year-old too young to go to the gym to strengthen his biceps? Is a sixty-year-old too old to walk three miles a day to strengthen his heart? Of course not. A muscle can be strengthened at any age. Strengthening exercises like these also lead to better health and a better sense of well-being, not to mention improved self-esteem.

The penis is no different. The PC muscle is a muscle, plain and simple. It works and responds like any other muscle, and it can be strengthened like any other muscle. And I've never seen a muscle that had a greater impact on a man's self-esteem.

Just a Few Minutes a Day

Mastering the techniques of male multiple orgasm is a snap once you are "PC-ready." And prepping your PC—getting it combat-ready—is simple. But you must be willing to stick with the program. That's why right now I'm going to ask you for a commitment.

I know how scary the word *commitment* can be to some guys, but this is one commitment you'll never regret. Every man who is willing to do the work can bring his PC muscle to a state of readiness within two to three weeks. Often it takes even less than that. All you need is a few minutes a day to work the program. That's right . . . just a few minutes a day. That's a whole lot less time than you probably spend in the gym right now working on every muscle in your body but the one that really counts.

I know you can do it. All you need to do is stay committed to the process. Remember, your ability to master the secrets of multiple orgasm depends on a strong PC muscle. So warm up those cold feet and say yes to a commitment that is bound to change your life.

Get Ready, Get Set . . .

We're almost ready to start. There's just one more piece of very important business we need to take care of. Within days of starting the exercise regimen in this book you are going to feel very different, and that's going to feel very good. But you are not the only one who is going to be feeling different. If you have a partner, your loving partner is going to be profoundly affected by all of the changes about to take place in your body and in your head. You need to attend to that, and you need to do that right now.

I know that you're probably feeling very excited about getting started. But it's important to make sure that your partner shares your enthusiasm. That's why, before I present any of the exercises, I must ask that you and your partner sit down and have a serious talk about the many ramifications of the journey you are *both* about to take. . . .

CHAPTER THREE

Talking to Your Partner About Male Multiple Orgasm

Making love to a multiorgasmic man is not business as usual. The intensity of responses and performance abilities can be quite startling to a woman who is used to a one-orgasm guy.

I'm not a big believer in surprises when it comes to sex. If there is a woman in your life right now, we need to make sure that she is every bit as prepared and every bit as committed to the process as you are. Sex doesn't happen in a vacuum. It happens between two people. Your needs are important, but the needs of the couple come first.

You will notice throughout the book that I have included guidelines for a partner in most of the exercises. Hopefully, your partner will want to follow those suggestions and take an active role in your development. Or maybe she'd rather just wait on the sidelines and reap the benefits at the end. That's fine too. It's up to both of you to decide what you're most comfortable with. But either way, your partner needs to know what's going on and you need to know that you have her support. I make sure that all of my clients have talked to their partners *before* they learn *any* of these techniques, and I must ask you to do the same thing. This conversation should not be taken lightly or given short shrift. A lot of changes are about to take place. Your attitude toward sex is about to change. Your attitude toward yourself is about to change. So are your abilities, your physiology, and your level of desire. Your partner has got a lot to reckon with.

If these changes are not discussed in advance, your efforts could backfire. If you try to keep the whole thing a secret, your partner could feel very left out. She might get confused, or insecure, or even angry. If she's used to Old Faithful, any kind of radical change could be quite disconcerting. She might even fear that you are having an affair and learning things from some other woman.

You *are* learning things from another woman, but this woman is a professional sex therapist whose only interest in you is that you learn techniques to enhance your relationship with your partner. The purpose of learning to become multiorgasmic is to bring you and your partner closer together. It is supposed to improve your relationship, not threaten it. You want your transformation to ignite your partner, not scare her. That's why I want you two to have a conversation, and I want you to have it as soon as possible after you have finished reading this book for the first time.

Talk to your partner. Tell her what you're up to, and don't withhold anything. Give her as much information as possible. Let her know why this is important to you. Tell her what your goals are, being sure to explain the benefits you can foresee for the relationship. It is very important that she knows you are doing this *for both of you*. Finally, tell her how important it is for you to have her support.

Male Multiple Orgasm Should Bring a Couple Together

Some women want to make love for hours at a time, whereas some are happiest when it's short and simple. The typical woman has different needs and desires on different days. What about your partner? What does she like, what does she want, and how might her needs vary from day to day and week to week? You need to know this information, and your conversation about embarking on this program is an ideal time to find out. Frankly, it's the only way both of you will fully benefit from your newfound talents. Otherwise, you may be doing all kinds of things that your partner simply isn't interested in.

Don't get me wrong. Your needs are important. But you must always remember that your partner's needs are equally important. There is nothing more unpleasant than a man who is just doing his thing, oblivious to what the woman really wants. Being a great lover means more than just tuning into your own body. Being a great lover means tuning into your partner's body too, and even more important, it means tuning into her mind.

The beauty of being multiorgasmic is that it gives you the kind of sexual flexibility you've never experienced before. For the first time, you can get tremendous pleasure without sacrificing any of your partner's needs. Your experience will be much more intense, but you're also going to help make hers more intense. You're doing wonderful things for yourself, but you also can attend to her in ways you never could before. No one has to make huge compromises or be shortchanged.

I have heard women complain about insensitive men who seem uninterested in what a woman really needs or men who couldn't go the distance. But I must tell you, I have never heard a woman complain about a man who could offer her whatever she desired.

When you and your partner have your talk, it is very important to talk about your needs, but it is probably even more important to talk about her needs. Let her tell you what she wants and what she doesn't want. Does anything make her uncomfortable? Is there anything she fears? Listen carefully to her answers, and don't assume anything. You may be surprised to discover that you know less about your partner than you think. This is a wonderful opportunity to express your caring and develop more closeness, and I encourage you to take advantage of it.

If your partner has a lot of questions about her specific role in your "training," reading through the book should give her the answers she is looking for. As you read through each partner exercise (some exercises do not require a partner), you will note that both the man's role and the woman's role are always clearly addressed. I highly recommend that *both* partners read the book, even if the woman is not going to participate in any of the exercises.

Every woman is different, and there is no way I can predict how your partner is going to respond to everything I present in this book. Personally, I hope she wants to make this a joint venture, so to speak. I say this because I know from experience that when a woman gets involved in the process it makes everything a lot more exciting for both partners. But, as I said before, it isn't necessary for a woman to help her man learn these new techniques; she only needs to be there at the finish line with a big smile on her face.

Did Your Partner Give You This Book?

If your partner gave you this book, your interest in male multiple orgasm will not be a surprise to her.

You probably already know that it is important to her that you improve your ability to prolong intercourse. But that doesn't mean that the two of you don't need to talk about it.

My one rule here is: *Don't assume anything*. Many of the issues in the preceding pages still need to be addressed. In addition, it's important for you to know what her expectations are, and to make sure that they are realistic.

If you feel pressured in any way, it's important to communicate this immediately to your partner. Even if you're a multiorgasmic man, performance pressure almost invariably interferes with sexual functioning, and that is something you do not want to happen. As I said before, the entire purpose of these techniques is to bring the two of you closer together, not drive you apart.

To the Women Reading This Book

Can we talk for a moment, woman to woman? If there's one thing that stops women from getting excited about the exercises in this book or getting involved, it's the fear that the whole process is going to be too mechanical. After all, how can a bunch of exercises be sexy? Some women feel uncomfortable about the whole idea of male multiple orgasm. Instead of looking forward to a richer sexual relationship, they fear that these techniques are going to turn their stud into a mechanical bull.

I need to dispel these concerns right now. Although doing exercises with a partner doesn't sound very sexy or very passionate, the techniques I am going to teach you unleash a level of passion and desire few couples ever experience. These exercises take a man into his body, not away from it. Even more important, they take a man into *your* body, not away from it. It is very sexy stuff. No longer feeling burdened by his anxieties or limitations, you will both be free to experience each other with far greater intensity than ever before. Now that doesn't sound so bad, does it?

There's one other thing we women need to talk about. As you read through the exercises in this book, you're going to notice pretty quickly that the vast majority of instructions are directed toward the male reader. This might make you feel a little bit left out, even if you're joining in for most of the exercises. Since it is the man who is learning to become multiorgasmic here and has most of the work to do, he requires the most instruction. I'm sure you can see the logic in that. But I don't want anyone to feel left out just because the one with the penis has the tougher job this time.

Remember that all of this is being done for *you*. Your partner is learning this to increase *your* pleasure and because he cares about *you*. You are the single most important motivation for his process. Period. But you are not a passive observer of his process, or a flexible love doll whose only purpose is to give your partner a female form on which to practice. You have a really important job here, and I mean that quite sincerely.

You can make or break these exercises for your partner because these are your exercises too. Your pleasure should never be compromised for his pleasure and your needs should never be compromised for his needs. The wonderful thing about learning these exercises is that it's an incredibly sensual, exciting experience for both partners. If it isn't, something is wrong, and you need to back up for a moment and consider where your experience got compromised.

Every man I teach says the same thing: the key ingredient to learning these exercises is an enthusiastic partner. A woman's excitement is contagious. It is the biggest turn-on a man could ask for. As I'm sure you all know from experience, a passive partner is deadly in *any* erotic encounter, and this erotic exercise regimen is no exception. If the woman isn't really excited about doing this with her partner, she shouldn't be doing it. It's that simple.

This is not one of those things you do for him, even though you really don't want to. When it comes to sex, it never makes sense to do anything for him if you're not enjoying it too. There should never be any suffering in a sexual relationship; there should only be pleasure and passion. If that sounds trite, forgive me, but it's true.

People who make big compromises in their sexual relationships are unhappy, and the relationship as a whole always suffers. That is something I do not want to encourage. I only want to make your relationship better, but I need your help and your trust to do it. If you honestly want to be a part of this exciting process, there is plenty for any woman to do. But the very first thing you need to do is let yourself have a wonderful time. Don't worry about him—he'll take care of himself. Just make sure *you* are always getting the most out of every experience.

As you do each exercise, think about how *you* might benefit the most. Make creative suggestions if you wish, and bring your own personality into the process. He'll love that.

If you are going to participate in these exercises, pay very close attention to your partner. Read through each exercise together before you begin so you know what to expect. Then try to really focus on your partner's experience in addition to focusing on your own. Try to feel his arousal as it rises and falls. Move the way he moves. Breathe the way he breathes. When he opens his eyes, open your eyes. If he moans, moan with him. If he falls asleep . . . if he falls asleep, poke him. Communicate as much as possible during each exercise. If the two of you stay really connected, you are going to feel most of what he is going through, and *it's going to be incredible for you too.* When two excited partners are deeply connected to each other, it makes for one hell of an amazing afternoon.

I need to ask you women one final favor. There are a few crucial moments in certain exercises when the man is instructed to stop moving. It is *very important* that the woman *stop with him.* Too much friction at the wrong moment might feel great, but it will probably end the exercise prematurely, if you know what I mean. I know it's going to get pretty exciting, and I know that sometimes it's really hard to suddenly stop what you are doing, but what you will quickly discover is that if you stop at the necessary moments, the payoff later on will be even bigger. So, keeping my one request in mind, go out there and have yourself a great time.

How to Use the Rest of This Book

All of the exercises in this book have been organized and presented with one goal in mind: to turn every single man who is reading this book into a multiorgasmic man. Every exercise is extremely important. Each serves a very specific purpose, and the order has been carefully chosen to make this step-by-step learning process as simple as possible. Though you will not actually have to complete every exercise in this book, I think it's a good idea to read through all of them.

You will notice later on that many of the exercises in this book are paired. In each pair, one exercise is designed for the man who is working with a partner and one is for the man who chooses to work alone. The exercises are labeled either "with a partner" or "solo" to make that clear.

In some cases I have presented the solo exercise first and in other cases I have presented the partner exercise first. This is because some exercises lend themselves more naturally to being tried first with a partner whereas others lend themselves more naturally to being tried first alone. But there is no right or wrong choice here, and I would not want to give that impression. Both exercises in each pair are totally valid, and it is up to you to choose the one you prefer.

It is my experience that most men prefer to mix it up a little bit, learning some techniques with their partners and learning others by themselves. That's perfectly okay. You can alternate any way you wish. You can even practice both exercises in a given pair if you want to, but it is not a requirement.

There are only two guidelines I ask you to follow:

GUIDELINE 1: Always do at least one of the two exercises in each pair. It doesn't matter whether you do the partner exercise or the solo exercise, but you *must* do one of them.

GUIDELINE 2: Please do the exercises in the order in which they are presented. The exercises build on each other, and you may get very frustrated if you try to skip around.

The easiest way to do these exercises is to read through each one before you begin. If you are working on a partner exercise, both of you should read through the exercise thoroughly. Discuss the exercise after you have read it. As I just explained to the women reading this book, both partners need to understand their roles in each exercise.

If either of you has any doubts, flush them out before you get started. Keep that line of communication open and clear. The more you talk now, the fewer complications you'll have once the lights are dimmed. Pace yourselves. Don't try to go through every exercise in a long weekend. Give yourselves weeks, or even months, to wander through the program. Learning to be multiorgasmic isn't anything like learning to play the violin. This process is going to be pleasurable from start to finish. You're not going to have to wait until you get to Carnegie Hall before you start enjoying yourself. The most important thing is that you take your time and keep the pressure off.

Keep Your Sex Safe!

As you read through the exercises in this book, you will notice that I have not specifically incorporated safe sex practices into the individual exercises. That's because I have written this book primarily for committed, monogamous couples who know each other to be safe from sexual risk.

I don't want to sound preachy here, but learning these techniques within the boundaries of a committed relationship is not only safer but more gratifying. Yet I realize that not all readers are currently in such a relationship. *If you are not in a committed, monogamous relationship yet wish to learn these techniques with a partner, it is crucial that you practice safe sex during every single exercise. Condoms must be used, even if you are not having intercourse!*

While it is true that condoms tend to desensitize the penis somewhat, they do not prohibit mastery of any of the techniques in the book. Many of my clients have used condoms throughout the training process with complete satisfaction, and the majority have told me that the condoms did not interfere at all. If you use condoms as a standard birth control practice, I also recommend using them in all of your exercises.

CHAPTER FOUR

The Complete PC Workout

I'm a big believer in foreplay, but enough is enough. It's time to get started. In this chapter you are going to learn the first set of simple exercises that will set the stage for taking control of your sexuality the way you have always imagined. Mastering them is the crucial first step on the path to a lifetime of pleasure and power as a multiorgasmic male. *The following three exercises are the most important exercises in the book. Please take them very seriously.* It is important to take your time, follow my instructions carefully, and try to be very thorough.

Unlike many of the exercises that follow, this first set of exercises is most easily accomplished on your own. If you have a partner who is waiting to work with you, let her know you'll be ready for her soon. You just need to prepare a few things. This should heighten her anticipation and make her all the more enthusiastic when it's time for her to join in.

So . . . let the games begin. Enjoy yourself! And don't forget: *PC power is ultimate power.*

Exercise 1: Hide and Seek

The very first thing you need to do is find your PC muscle. For some men this is very simple—you probably knew where to find it the moment I mentioned it. You may even be squeezing it right now.

But many men are completely unfamiliar with the muscles in this area of the body. All of the individual muscles close to the groin—buttocks, abdomen, thighs, and PC—may feel the same. They might all feel like one big muscle mass. That needs to change right now. Here is the simplest way to find your PC muscle and isolate it from all the others.

First, gently place one or two fingers right behind your testicles. Pretend that you are urinating. Now try to stop the flow. That muscle you just used to turn off the flow from the bladder is your PC muscle. Did you feel it tightening? Maybe you also noticed that your penis and testicles "jumped" a little when you flexed your PC.

It is very important that your stomach muscles and thigh muscles remain relaxed. Did they get tense too? Try again. This time focus just on the PC.

TROUBLESHOOTING TIP: You are not trying to get an erection here, and you do not need an erection to exercise the PC. So relax, and let your penis respond naturally to these exercises.

Exercise 2: Squeeze Play (three to five minutes a day)

Now that you've found your PC muscle, here is your next exercise: Three times a day, flex the PC twenty times. Hold it for one or two seconds each time, then release. That's it. Twenty squeezes, three times a day. I know it sounds simple, but words cannot express how important this exercise is.

You do not need to keep your finger on the PC during these exercises. You should be able to feel it move internally. If you don't, or if you're not sure, then keep your finger on the PC the first few times you do your exercises.

Breathe normally during this exercise. Like any other muscle-building exercise, proper breathing is always important. You don't want to hold your breath.

I want you to repeat this exercise *three times a day, every day, for three weeks.* A consistent exercise regimen is the most effective way to maximize the strengthening of your PC muscle in the shortest amount of time. And it's worth every moment.

ROAD TRIP

I know this sounds like a commercial, but these PC exercises are easy and can be done anywhere—in the car, at the beach, or while sitting at your desk. Many men tell me that half the fun of prepping is being able to do it in broad daylight in front of city hall with no fear of being arrested for indecent exposure! Okay, I'm exaggerating. But men do tell me that prepping the PC is a lot of fun.

Now that you've isolated your PC muscle and learned how to squeeze, you might want to take your act on the road. Do you ride the bus to work? A perfect opportunity. Long line at the bank? Why not. Having lunch alone? Not anymore. Of course, you may prefer to keep your exercise regimen safe at home, but you have many options.

Two PC Pitfalls

These exercises are not hard, but there are two common mistakes men make when they start these exercises that you need to be aware of before we go any further:

MISTAKE 1: *Doing too many reps.* I know you're feeling very enthusiastic right now, but there is such a thing as overdoing it. The PC muscle can get sore like any other muscle. You may have already discovered this on your own. Go slow at first, as you would when you start any other exercise for the first time, and let the muscle build. You can pour it on later.

MISTAKE 2: *Failing to isolate the PC.* The PC is a small group of muscles, which need to be isolated from the many larger muscles close by during your exercises. As I said before, it is important that your stomach, upper thighs, and buttocks are all completely relaxed when you are working out the PC. They should not be moving.

Are you having difficulty isolating the PC from other muscles? Many men have this problem when they try these exercises for the first time. Not to worry. If you can't stop yourself from tensing other muscles during your PC exercises, you simply need to exhaust these muscles first so they don't interfere with your new exercise regimen.

Let's say you have a tendency to tense your stomach muscles during your PC workout. What you need to do is tense and untense your stomach muscles at least ten or twenty times before you begin your PC exercises. That should tire them out enough so they don't get in the way. The same applies for buttock, thigh, and groin muscles. If you have to work these muscles really hard before you get to work on your PC, that's okay. Do thirty or forty reps if twenty isn't enough. This may sound like a lot of work, but you're not going to have to do this for the rest of your life—just for a couple of days.

Once you have really isolated your PC, your muscle "confusion" should dissolve, leaving you free to devote your full attention to working the program. With that in mind, let us now return to our regularly scheduled program, already in progress.

Exercise 3: The Big Squeeze (two to three minutes a day)

Have you done your reps three times a day for the last three weeks? Good. Now you're ready to learn what I call "The Big Squeeze" (a.k.a. "The Power Squeeze" or "The Death Grip"). I want you to keep doing your twenty quick squeezes, three times a day. But now you're going to add ten really *slow* squeezes. This is what you do. Take five seconds to slowly squeeze your PC as tight as you can. Now hold the tension for a full five seconds, if possible. Finally, release the tension gradually over the next five seconds. You should be able to feel yourself really working the muscle.

This might be a bit difficult at first. You may only be able to do one or two fifteen-second squeezes before you tire. That's okay. But try to eventually work up to ten full repetitions, each taking ten to fifteen seconds. It may take you a few days, or even a few weeks, to get there. That's okay. It's more important that you don't push yourself too hard. You're not training to be an American Gladiator. Just enjoy the process and keep squeezing.

Meet Early and Meet Often

The PC workout is like any other workout. The harder you work, the faster and more impressive the results. The great thing about the PC is that, unlike some muscles, it responds so quickly to being exercised. No matter how intense or casual your workout is, you won't have to spend months and months before you notice a difference. As you will soon see, the PC workout brings immediate gratification. Still, you need to be thorough.

There are several steps to becoming multiorgasmic, but building up the PC is the crucial first step. Don't give it short shrift. There are no deadlines here, no clocks to punch, and no boss to report to. The most important thing is to get the job done. Are you one of those people who takes the new VCR out of the box and tries to make it work without reading a single page of the instruction manual? I'm the same way. But this kind of attitude simply won't work when it comes to mastering the techniques for male multiple orgasm.

My grandmother used to say to me, "You can't run in the Olympics until you've learned to tie your sneakers." Listen to grandma. Take it one step at a time and take your time on every step. You'll be at the finish line before you know it, being hugged by your biggest fan. Meanwhile, that will give us some time to talk a little bit more about the miracle of male multiple orgasm.

CHAPTER FIVE

Male Multiple Orgasm— The Secret Revealed

What exactly *is* male multiple orgasm? Is it anything like a regular orgasm or is it completely different? Is it better than a regular orgasm? Is it a lot of work? Is it different from female multiple orgasm? Can any man have one? Questions, questions, questions. Your head is probably spinning from all of the questions you have at this very moment. And let us not forget the most important one of all: *How do you do it?*

Male Multiple Orgasm: My Definition

A multiorgasmic man, quite simply, is a man who can have two or more orgasms in a row without resting. He does not experience any significant down time between his orgasms. By "down time," I mean a refractory period in between orgasms when the penis is not easily aroused. A multiorgasmic man is able to maintain his erection, even though he has already had an orgasm, and continue making love from orgasm to orgasm. Unlike most "normal" men, a multiorgasmic man does not lose his ability to stay erect after his first orgasm. He can continue to a second or even a third or fourth orgasm without resting.

This is not the same as having two or more orgasms in an afternoon of lovemaking with periods of rest or breaks in between. The multiorgasmic man does not need a rest. He might want to, and he certainly can, if he or his partner wishes, but he doesn't *have* to stop. He is capable of continuing to make love *immediately* after orgasm.

How Is This Possible?

There are some men, particularly young men, who are just plain lucky. These guys are naturals. Their physiology is such that they don't lose their erections after orgasm, or they regain their erections so quickly that intercourse is barely interrupted. Men like this are "born" multiorgasmic. Maybe there was a time in your life when you were this lucky too. But chances are, those days are gone. Well, the good news is that you don't have to be lucky anymore to be multiorgasmic. There is another way to acquire this ability, and it works regardless of your age, your experience, or your God-given talents.

The secret to becoming multiorgasmic is actually quite simple. The secret, for most men who have mastered the ability, lies in learning to have a complete orgasm without ejaculating. That's right, a full, powerful orgasm—or two, or three, or more— *with no ejaculation.* Without ejaculation there is no refractory period—no down time. That means there is no significant loss of erection, leaving you free to continue having intercourse until you reach the point where you are ready to have an orgasm *with* simultaneous ejaculation.

Orgasm Without Ejaculation! . . . Am I Crazy?

Now, I know that this may not sound as simple as I say it is. There's a really good chance that at this moment it all sounds very weird, or even impossible. I realize that as far as most men are concerned, there is no such thing as an orgasm without ejaculation. It's a package deal, like thunder and lightning, right? Wrong. This may be hard to believe, but as most sex therapists will confirm, *orgasm and ejaculation in males are two separate things.* Yes, they typically occur together, and yes, it *feels* as though they are a package deal. But the physiological reality is that they are not inseparable. It is possible to have a full orgasm without a simultaneous ejaculation, and therein lies the key to becoming multiorgasmic. Learn how to separate them, and you're on your way.

I know that this news isn't mind-boggling for every man who is reading this book right now. Many men have stumbled onto this accidentally. In fact, there may already have been an occasion or two in *your* life when you actually experienced the sensations of orgasm without having an ejaculation.

At the time, you may not have thought much of it, or you might have found it confusing. Most men who experience this unintentionally think that it's an accident or some strange quirk. Many worry that something might be wrong with them, but very few men think of it as an experience worth recapturing, let alone perfecting. If you did, you probably wouldn't be reading this book right now—you'd be out there doing it. But believe me, I know hundreds of men who would gladly tell you that a nonejaculatory orgasm is an experience worth recapturing and worth perfecting. These men will also tell you that if you've never had a nonejaculatory orgasm, you need to start. And that's what you're going to do, with my help.

Meet James, a Multiorgasmic Man

I'd like to introduce you to James, one of several multiorgasmic men you'll hear about, a man who has been practicing these techniques for almost eight years. I want you to read James's story first because his method of having multiple orgasms most closely resembles the style we focus on in this book. You may not necessarily have intercourse for the same length of time as James does, but the techniques you use will not differ significantly.

When James and his partner Sharon make love, he typically takes ten minutes or more before he has an orgasm. He starts intercourse slowly and lets his arousal build. Then the instant before he is about to ejaculate, he thrusts deeply into Sharon and squeezes the muscle that runs from the base of the penis to the area behind his testicles. This allows him to have a full orgasm—including rapid heart rate, muscle contractions, and that incredible sensation of release—*without an ejaculation*.

James maintains his erection, continues to make love, and has two to four more orgasms this way. When he wants to stop making love, he has a final orgasm and ejaculates. James is able to do this because he has achieved good control of the pelvic muscles that spasm when a man ejaculates.

James usually lets his partner's desires guide him. If Sharon wants to have intercourse for a long time, he simply delays his ejaculation until she's had all she wants. In the meantime, he may have three or four *full* orgasms. If Sharon wants to make it a shorter evening, James complies happily. Some nights are marathons and some nights are quickies. The important thing is, it's their decision.

Alan's Story

Alan used to have one quick orgasm when he made love and then call it a night. Today, however, Alan is a two-orgasm guy. When he is making love with his wife, Alan's first orgasm tends to come on rather quickly—within five minutes or less. But Alan has learned to contract his PC muscle at just the right moment before his climax, and this completely suppresses his ejaculation. Alan calls this first orgasm his "dry" orgasm. This is usually his most powerful orgasm, but it is just the beginning of his lovemaking.

With orgasm number one out of the way, Alan "settles in" for the slow journey to orgasm number two. What Alan likes to do here is time his second orgasm so that it occurs with, or just after, his wife's orgasm. Alan and his wife find this to be extremely gratifying for both of them. Alan's wife tends to need prolonged intercourse before she can climax, which is why she was so enthusiastic about helping Alan learn these techniques.

Alan and his wife have developed a set of non-verbal signals (winks, nods, squeezes, etc.) that help them get their timing right. When it is time for their mutual climax, Alan just relaxes all of the muscles he tensed the first time, and has a second full orgasm, complete with ejaculation. Alan says, "The first one is for me. . . . The second one is for both of us."

The Multiorgasmic Male: Some Variations on a Theme

The exercises in this book will teach you what I believe to be the simplest, most effective way for a man to become multiorgasmic. But that's just the beginning. Once you have mastered these techniques, you may go on to develop your own unique style. In the many years I have worked with men, I have seen all kinds of interesting variations on the theme of multiple orgasm. For example, while most men achieve multiple orgasms by delaying ejaculation, some are able to have partial or even complete ejaculations without losing their erections. While most men spread out their orgasms through a prolonged session of lovemaking, some men experience all of their orgasms in rapid-fire succession.

There is no predicting what you will be capable of or what will feel best to you. Your body is unique, and it will respond in a unique way. Maybe you will develop some variation I have yet to see. Wouldn't that be great? Drop me a line if you do, because I'm always interested in hearing about new things.

I want to introduce you to two other multiorgasmic men whose styles are quite different from James and Alan's so that you can get a sense of the many possibilities that lie ahead. As you read their stories, remember that as different as these styles may seem, all four men started their multiorgasmic "careers" with the same basic techniques.

Bob Can Ejaculate More Than Once Without Losing His Erection

Bob has a very different way of reaching multiple orgasms. When Bob makes love to his wife he tends to begin by thrusting very vigorously and often ejaculates within about five minutes. However, after ejaculating, he has learned to maintain both his erection and his arousal, and he continues to thrust slowly. Within minutes he is able to have another complete ejaculation and orgasm, as strong as the first. If he chooses, he can continue making love in this fashion, having as many as five or six orgasms and ejaculations within an hour.

Bob's ability to extend his lovemaking in this fashion gives his wife Janice the extra time she needs to reach her own peak. This is something she was unable to do with Bob before he developed this ability. Janice and Bob used to compensate for their incompatibility with oral sex or manual manipulation, but Janice always felt somewhat disappointed that she was unable to reach her orgasm through straight intercourse. Today, Janice is a very satisfied woman.

Bob's style of multiple orgasm is called multi-ejaculation, and it is a more advanced and difficult technique to master than James's. What Bob has learned to do is shorten his refractory period, thereby shortening the length of time it takes him to become aroused again after he has ejaculated.

John's Pattern Resembles Many Women's Experience

When making love, John usually thrusts for approximately ten or fifteen minutes until he has a very strong orgasm with a partial ejaculation. After this, his penis becomes even more sensitive, adding to his pleasure. His erection does not dissipate and he continues to thrust vigorously. Then, within a short period of time, he experiences a series of smaller orgasms, almost like aftershocks.

John's experience is most similar to a type of multiple orgasm many women experience. This style of multiple orgasm is not uncommon for multiorgasmic men. I have heard many stories of men who developed this technique on their own by actually mimicking the breathing patterns and muscle movements of multiorgasmic women. The interesting thing about John is that he no longer has to try to make any of this happen. He has conditioned his body so well that this aftershock response is now completely automatic, happening every time he has an orgasm.

Four "A" Students

James, Bob, John, and Alan are all multiorgasmic men, although, as you can see, the experience of having multiple orgasms is somewhat different for each of them. But James, Bob, John, and Alan have something else in common. None of them were naturally multiorgasmic. All of them learned to have multiple orgasms by using the exact same techniques presented in this book!

These four men have still one more thing in common: James, Alan, Bob, and John were all my "students." I saw each one move from being a single-orgasmic beginner to a multiorgasmic graduate. I am proud of them all, and they are all proud of themselves.

When a man turns to a sex therapist for help, his sexual functioning is usually a source of great distress. These four men were all struggling when I met them for the first time, and look at what they can do now. Just imagine the possibilities that lie ahead for a man like you who may already be fairly comfortable with his ability to perform.

"I Want to Believe This, But . . . "

I sense that you are very close to becoming a believer. Once you know the secret formula for male multiple orgasms, it all begins to make perfect sense, doesn't it? But I wouldn't be surprised if you're wondering right now how something so extraordinary and so simple could go unnoticed for so long. After all, the sexual revolution ended years ago. How could we have missed a phenomenon like male multiple orgasm? If such a thing is as easy for any man to achieve as I say it is, why isn't every guy in America doing it? And why aren't you doing it right now? These are really important questions. And I have some surprising answers:

FACT: **Male multiple orgasm is nothing new.** Eastern cultures, for example, have been aware of male multiple orgasm and nonejaculatory orgasm (NEO) for many years, and it is not difficult to find references

to it in their tantric literature and historical literature. High up on mountaintops in faraway lands,
both men and women have been having a good old
time for a long, long time.

FACT: **Male multiple orgasm is well documented in
professional publications.** Knowledge of this phenomenon has not been restricted to a handful of
enlightened souls living on distant shores. References
to male multiple orgasm, some dating back as far as
the 1930s, can be found in numerous books and journal articles available at most college libraries right
here in the good old United States.

A Quick History Lesson

The earliest news of the existence of male multiple
orgasm was not well received in this country. Quite
the contrary, when it was first mentioned in the scientific literature in the 1930s and early 1940s, it was
viewed as dysfunctional, or even pathological. In
other words, most professionals believed that it
only happened to a man if there was something
wrong with his equipment. Given the prevailing
attitude at the time, it is no wonder that the whole
thing got very little attention.

Then, in 1948, Alfred Kinsey's groundbreaking
book, *Sexual Behavior in the Human Male*, was published. In the book, Kinsey clearly noted that several
of the "normal" men he studied reported having
more than one ejaculation with the same erection.
Others reported experiencing the sensations of
orgasm without ejaculation, and some reported
more than one climax with each act of intercourse.

Now you would think that news like this would have spread like wildfire, but it didn't. Although the professional community became more accepting of the concept, the standard belief was that "either you have it or you don't." In other words, men didn't *become* multiorgasmic: either they were born that way or they weren't born that way. And that was that. It wasn't until the 1970s that professionals began to consider a third possibility: that male multiple orgasm could actually be learned. That's when the real fun started. Ever since then, many open-minded sex therapists, myself and my colleagues included, have been working long and hard (no jokes please) to develop and refine a number of valid techniques that any man could learn. Though we all like to argue about whose methods are best, there is one thing we all agree on: *it can be done.*

Well, that ends our little history lesson. It's the nineties and you're a lucky guy. Today, all of the necessary techniques exist for men to become multiorgasmic. All you need to do now is the work. If you want to learn more about the evolution of this exciting and important discovery, I suggest you take a look at some of the articles I've listed at the end of the book in Appendix 1.

"Are You Sure There Isn't a Catch?"

If you're not a multiorgasmic male, you might be inclined to think that a nonejaculatory orgasm wouldn't feel all that fabulous—that it might be a bit feeble, relatively speaking. I can understand why it's probably hard to imagine that an orgasm without an ejaculation could possibly feel as intense as the old reliable orgasm/ejaculation combo. But have I got a surprise for you. More than half the men I have spoken to report that their nonejaculatory orgasms are more powerful than any traditional orgasm they ever had. That's right . . . not just *as* good as a traditional orgasm . . . better! When you hear these men explain their experiences, it begins to make sense. Look, for example, at what these four men have to say:

> The nonejaculatory orgasm is actually more intense
> in some ways because you are planning it, leading
> up to it, and you know it is going to happen. In my
> "previous sex life," even though every orgasm had
> an ejaculation with it, sometimes the orgasm was
> not very strong because I wasn't totally expecting it.
> Or I was actually trying to hold it back so it got sort
> of muffled. Sometimes I would actually have an
> ejaculation without an orgasm. That was very
> unpleasant.
>
> —*Frank, age 58*

> With the buildup I need to have more than one
> orgasm, the crown of my penis gets extremely sen-
> sitive and tingly. If I stretch it out long enough, my
> first orgasm feels like the top of my head is blowing
> off.
>
> —*Thomas, age 41*

> I don't have multiple orgasms or nonejaculatory
> orgasms every time I have sex. Sometimes I have
> sex just as a release or a way to be close with my
> partner before I fall asleep. But I have sex with

nonejaculatory orgasms when I really want to take some time and have an intense experience.

—*Edward, age 27*

When I first heard about this I thought there is no way that having an orgasm without an ejaculation could feel the same. I thought it would feel disappointing, or like I'd missed something. But it's not like that at all. Now I am really feeling what is happening during orgasm. Before, it would happen so fast that I wasn't even aware of what I was feeling.

—*Justin, age 33*

Are you feeling a little more convinced? I have heard comments like these over and over and over again. I'm not surprised anymore, but I'm always impressed. I bet you're impressed too, but I bet you're also getting anxious. We can talk and talk and talk about the wonders of male multiple orgasm, but there comes a time when you've got to get down to business. Every day, more and more men are becoming multiorgasmic, and I think it's time you had your chance.

CHAPTER SIX

Learning to Touch, Learning to Feel

The material in this chapter always reminds me of two of my very first clients, Andrew and Eleanor. Andrew and Eleanor came to my office because Eleanor was extremely distressed by Andrew's lack of sensitivity during intercourse. Eleanor said that having sex with Andrew was like having a drill on top of her. She complained that he was like a robot, pounding away, not even noticing when her head hit against the headboard of the bed. Andrew admitted how detached he felt from his body during sex. He also admitted to being quite anxious. Andrew felt that if he didn't perform in exactly this fashion either he would lose his erection or Eleanor would lose interest.

The thought of slowing down and experiencing intercourse "in the moment" was totally foreign to Andrew. At first, it was also a bit anxiety provoking. I knew that Andrew needed to slow down and learn to appreciate his own body before he could appreciate his wife. That's why I began his therapy by teaching him certain sensate focus exercises, which he could do with Eleanor, or by himself, that would help him experience his own body. In this chapter, I'm going to teach you many of these same exercises. This is not to imply that I think all men are as out of touch with their bodies as Andrew was. These techniques are invaluable for any man, regardless of his current level of awareness.

Men, as we all know, tend to be very target oriented. They want to get it up and get it in. As far as most women are concerned, this makes for very uninteresting sex. But it also makes it extremely difficult for a man to have a multiple orgasm. This chapter will help you develop a greater appreciation for the changes in your physiology as they are continually taking place during arousal. It will help you more fully experience your most pleasurable bodily sensations as they are happening, and set the stage for prolonging and intensifying each of these sensations.

Getting sensitized to your own arousal process is really important if you want to become multiorgasmic. A good pilot doesn't just know how to fly; a good pilot knows the workings of the airplane inside and out. A virtuoso doesn't just play an instrument; a virtuoso has an intimate relationship with the instrument. The same thing applies to sex. It's not enough to just own a penis. You need to be intimate with the many nuances of your own sexual response if you want to learn the special techniques in the following chapters and master the art of male multiple orgasm.

What Exactly Is Sensate Focus?

Sensate focus techniques are structured sensual touching exercises designed by sex therapists to help men and women focus on, appreciate, and control the moment-to-moment experiences of contact, arousal, and release. These well-established techniques create a level of physiological awareness that leads to extraordinary control over the different phases of excitement, orgasm, and ejaculation.

We are going to use sensate focus techniques in most of our exercises. These are not sex acts. They are very loving, very pleasurable ways of making contact with a partner. Arousal is not the goal here.

Orgasm is not the goal. Your only goal is full appreciation of the sensations you are about to experience.

Sensate Focus Takes You into Your Body

For many people, sex in an ongoing relationship has a way of becoming a bit routine. Are you concerned because something that was once so charged and passionate has lost a lot of its punch? Are you always searching for new fantasies to keep the fire alive? Well, sensate focus is going to change all of that.

I think that one of the main reasons sex loses its spark is because of the way we all rush through the process. As far as I'm concerned, most people are having sex too darn fast. It seems as though everyone is in such a hurry to get to the point of orgasm that they are missing all of the wonderful things that happen to their body, and to their partner's body, along the way. If you want to make your sex life more exciting and more erotic, I think the very first thing you need to do is stop rushing. And that's where sensate focus comes in.

Sensate focus techniques slow you down. They take you into your body and into your partner's body in ways you have probably never experienced before. I think fantasies are wonderful, but fantasies tend to take us out of our bodies and into our heads. Sometimes, I think that can be the wrong direction. Personally, I think that what we really need to enhance our experience of sex is not more fantasy, but a much bigger dose of reality. Sensate focus gives you that reality. It focuses your attention and your energy and lets you appreciate every single erotic nuance of your arousal and your partner's arousal. To me, that's the ultimate aphrodisiac.

Play by the Rules

Before we begin, you need to know the three rules of sensate focus:

RULE 1: Pay attention to exactly where you are touching or where you are being touched. Try to stay as focused as possible.

RULE 2: Stay in the here and now. Don't think about what happened last week or what could happen next Thursday. Try to let go of anything that is not happening at this very moment.

RULE 3: Don't put any pressure on yourself. If you're working with a partner, don't put any pressure on her either. Sex therapists call this "nondemand interaction." I will call the sensate focus exercises "demand-free" or "pressure-free" exercises. There are no grades here, no good and bad, no right or wrong, just touching and being touched.

Preparing for the Exercises

From this point forward, I recommend you do all of the exercises in the book in a quiet room that is free from distractions. You are going to need a comfortable bed (you may prefer a comfortable chair for the solo exercises). You are also going to need some K-Y jelly, baby oil, massage oil, cream, or other lubricant. Be sure to use a lubricant that does not irritate the genitals—for women, K-Y jelly is usually the safest choice. Keep a clean towel handy. If you use condoms, have them by the bedside within easy reach.

You may find it helpful to have a clock to keep you from completely losing track of the time. If there is a telephone in the room, turn it off. If there are children in the house, they should be sound asleep or with a babysitter. The room should be lit according to your preferences, but I don't recommend playing any music. You need to focus as much as possible on the sensations you are about to experience.

If you were learning these techniques at our offices, the setup would be no different. We provide a quiet room with a bed, lubricants, clock, towel, etc. There is no special equipment that is required.

Learning the Genital Caress

There are many different sensate focus techniques. For the purposes of this book, however, there is only one technique that you need to learn: the genital caress. You can learn the sensate focus genital caress with a partner (Exercise 4) or by yourself (Exercise 5). You are going to need about one hour for Exercise 4 and thirty minutes for Exercise 5.

Exercise 4: Touch of Heaven (with a partner)

In this exercise, one partner will play the *active* role while the other plays the *passive* role. Then you will switch in the middle so no one feels shortchanged.

Let's say that the woman is going to be the passive partner first. The first thing she needs to do is lie on her back and get very comfortable. She needs to take her time and get completely relaxed. This exercise does not begin until the passive partner is completely relaxed.

As the active partner, you are going to start slowly, gently stroking the front of her body for about fifteen or twenty minutes. The style of touching is called a caress. When you caress, you touch in a very, very slow, focused fashion. Because this is a genital caress, your stroking is going to focus primarily on her genitals, though it does not have to be limited to her genitals.

Slowly start to caress her genitals with your fingers or mouth, touching both the outside and inside of her vagina. Use lots of lubrication. Focus intently on the areas you are touching. Pay careful attention to what they feel like and what they look like. Absorb yourself in those sensations. Remember that this is a demand-free exercise. You are not touching to please her or to turn her on. You are touching to please *you*. That takes the pressure off her and it also takes the pressure off you.

All your partner needs to do is lie still, relax, and feel her sensations. She should stay completely passive, with her eyes closed. She shouldn't move. She should not try to reciprocate. She should not talk unless you are making her uncomfortable. She needs only to let herself feel your touch. If she gets distracted, she needs to gently bring her focus back to where you are touching her. If you notice her body getting tense, lightly pat her on the leg as a signal for her to relax. Try to stay as focused as possible, deeply absorbed in touching her and the way that feels. If your mind starts wandering, you need to gently refocus your mind on the caress. It doesn't matter how many times your mind strays. All that matters is that each time you recognize the shift, you bring yourself back to the exercise.

This is a wonderful technique for learning to relax and connect to your feelings. Your only goal is to get as much pleasure as possible for yourself while your partner is getting as much pleasure as possible for herself. If you find yourself getting mechanical or getting bored with your caressing, slow down. Chances are, you aren't letting yourself really be in the moment.

TROUBLESHOOTING TIP: If you start rubbing your partner's clitoris or trying to turn her on in some way, she will be able to feel the shift in your intentions. She is playing the passive role and is not supposed to respond in any way. So don't try to change the rules. Stick with the program.

Now it's your turn. Once you've played the active role for about twenty minutes, you are ready to switch roles. (Of course, you can take longer if you wish.) This time, the man will be taking the *passive* role.

Lie down comfortably on your back with your legs slightly spread. Let your arms rest at your sides, or place them under your head. Once you have settled into a position, try not to change it.

Your partner will spend the next twenty or so minutes caressing the front of your body, concentrating primarily on caressing your genitals. I recommend she uses baby oil or some other lubricant you both like. She can caress you with her hands, with her mouth, or with both.

Your job is to stay focused on her touch, and how it feels. Don't move around and don't talk. Let your partner explore the feeling of touching your penis and scrotum.

It does not matter whether or not you get an erection. A soft penis should feel as good to her as a hard penis, just different. She is only focusing on the sensation of touching you, not on your arousal (and not on hers). If you do get an erection, it is very important to understand that you don't have to do anything with it. All you need to do right now is enjoy the sensations of your own arousal.

TROUBLESHOOTING TIP: Make sure your partner knows that her goal is not to turn you on. All she is supposed to do is touch you in a way that *feels good to her*.

Don't flex your PC muscle during this exercise. Don't hold your breath. Just close your eyes, relax, and focus on her caresses. If you become very aroused and you ejaculate, that's okay. Just let your partner wipe you off and continue her caress. The important thing is that you don't try to force anything.

If your partner senses that you are tensing up, she should signal you to relax by gently tapping you on the leg. The only time you should talk to her is if she is doing something that makes you uncomfortable. Otherwise, just release yourself into the moment and enjoy the sensations.

If you find yourself drifting off, gently bring your focus back to where your partner is touching you. It doesn't matter how often you drift. Just practice bringing yourself back into the moment.

If you don't have a partner, or if you prefer to practice by yourself, the sensate focus genital caress is still quite pleasurable. It is important to remember that this is not a masturbation exercise. It is a way of experiencing the many rich sensations of your own arousal. Ejaculation is not a goal. If it happens, that's fine, but you are not trying to *make* it happen. Your goal is simply to create and experience as much sensation in your penis as possible.

Exercise 5: Alone at Last (solo)

Lie on your back, close your eyes, and get very comfortable (you may prefer to sit in a comfortable chair). Using plenty of lubrication, slowly, gently touch yourself in a caressing way. You may want to start by touching your nipples or thighs, since both are probably quite sensitive. Then slowly move to the genitals. Once you begin caressing your penis, do not use a masturbation stroke. Do not try to turn yourself on. Explore every crease and fold in the genital area. Take your time.

Remember that the most important thing is to stay as relaxed as possible and focused on the here and now. You are not trying to *do* anything except enjoy the sensations. If you have an erection, that's fine. If you don't, that's fine too. But you should not be trying to give yourself one. This is a pressure-free exercise. All you want to do is experience the richness of your own arousal. If your mind starts to wander, gently bring your focus back to the sensations you're experiencing in the moment. This may happen several times. That's okay. Just keep bringing your focus back to the exercise.

TROUBLESHOOTING TIP: If you have thoughts like, "I wonder if I'm really hard," or "I wonder if I could give myself an orgasm," you are thinking about your performance. That means you're putting subtle pressure on yourself. Just stay with the sensations. That's your only goal.

I suggest you do this exercise for at least twenty minutes, if not longer. Thirty minutes is ideal. Sometimes, in the absence of a partner, there is a tendency to rush everything. This defeats the whole purpose of sensate focus. Remember that the emphasis is on sensuality, not sexuality. Some men feel a bit self-conscious during this exercise. This is very normal, especially if you are a man who does not masturbate often, or someone who tends to rush to the point of climax. Don't be concerned. Your discomfort should ease over time.

It Sure Feels Good, But . . .

The sensate focus genital caress feels pretty terrific. That's reason enough to learn it. From this point on, almost every exercise in this book begins with this caress. That's another good reason to learn it. But why is it so important?

The sensate focus genital caress lets you pay attention to your sensations without getting distracted. It lets you focus. It lets you stay in the here and now. And it keeps the pressure off you and off your partner. You need to be able to do all of these things to master the art of male multiple orgasm.

We can talk and talk about the many benefits of the sensate focus genital caress. But you need some experience actually *feeling* it. That's why I've included the above exercises. So enjoy yourself, repeat them as many times as you like, but remember that the pleasure you're getting right now is only one of the payoffs.

CHAPTER SEVEN

Aroused and Aware

Y ou have to know where you are to know where you're going. Unfortunately most men have a very limited awareness of their own sexual responses and they don't always know what they are feeling or experiencing at the moment. They know that something pleasurable is happening, but they don't know exactly what that something is. They know that they're aroused, that's for sure, but they aren't in touch with the subtleties of their own experience. This is very limiting, both for the man and for his partner.

This chapter teaches a man how to know what is happening to his body during the various stages of arousal. He will learn how to listen to what his body is telling him, and how to work with those signals to maximize both his pleasure and the pleasure he is giving his partner.

How Aroused Are You?

Ask the average man if he's feeling aroused and what does he say? "Yes" or "No." Ask him to describe his arousal and what does he say? Not a whole lot more. But talk to a multiorgasmic man about his arousal and you're having a very different conversation. Multiorgasmic men are masters of their own arousal. They know the nuances of their erotic experience and take advantage of their sensitivity to prolong and magnify that experience. Ask a multiorgasmic man to describe his arousal and he'll give you at least five pages, single spaced. He might even throw in a poem.

Sexual arousal is actually a very complex and sophisticated process. There are many levels of arousal, each having its own distinct sensations and intensity. Some shifts are subtle, some are profound, but it is not a black or white thing. It's a lot more like a rainbow. What we are going to focus on right now is learning to recognize and appreciate these different colors of the rainbow by becoming more aware of the subtle differences of each one.

Once you are sensitized to your many levels of arousal, you will have a much more intimate relationship with your own body. That becomes really important when you start working with your body toward your first multiple orgasm. If multiple orgasm is your goal, being aroused is not enough. You must be aroused *and* aware. It's like learning to write music. Everything may sound nice to your ear, but it's hard to write a song until you know all of the notes on the scale. The more you refine your ear, the easier it gets. Sharps and flats are more subtle, but they are extremely important too.

By the time you've completed the exercises in this chapter, you are going to know the various levels of your own arousal the way a composer knows the notes on the scale. To make this easier, we are going to establish a scale of our own: an arousal scale.

Learning the Scales

Our arousal scale is going to be a very simple scale that goes from one to ten, with Level 1 being the lowest level of arousal and Level 10 being the highest.

Let's begin with Level 1. Level 1 is your baseline. What does it feel like? Let me give you an example. It's Saturday afternoon on a hot summer day. You've just finished your lunch and you're thinking of doing the laundry. Your dog wants to go for a walk and your car needs a wash. There isn't a sexual thought in your head. You are not experiencing any arousal whatsoever. None. Zero. Nada. Get the picture? At that moment, you are at Level 1.

Let's now jump to Level 10. That's an easy one. Level 10 is orgasm. The Big "O." The end of the road.

Great. Now all we need to do is establish everything in between. A Level 2 or Level 3 is that slight twinge sensation a man gets at the base of his penis as he begins to get aroused. The beast within has started to stir at the first whiff of something exciting in the air. It's subtle, but it's there.

Next comes Level 4. That's a steady, low level of arousal. It's more than a twinge now . . . you're feeling good. Still, you could stop without much difficulty. But that's going to change soon. At Level 5 and Level 6 your arousal is already substantial. Now you're really into it. Once you've reached these levels, you don't want to think about stopping. You're feeling *too* good now. By the time you get to Level 7 or Level 8, you will feel your heart pounding and your face may flush. If you had to talk you would probably sound out of breath. Level 9 is intense. You aren't far from the top now . . . you are very close to orgasm. At Level 9, the outside world is very far away, and there isn't much that could stop you now.

Just short of Level 10 is a very crucial point I call "the point of no return." It is commonly referred to as "the point of inevitability." You may not know the name, but I bet you know the feeling. It's that point at which it becomes clear that you are about to have an orgasm. The point of inevitability is reached through a series of physiological changes in the body, but it is subjectively experienced as a psychological turning point.

Once you've hit the point of inevitability, there is no going back. Your body is committed to having that orgasm. The sky could fall in and worlds could collide, but it doesn't matter as far as you are concerned. The big one is on the way.

On our 1 to 10 scale, this "point of no return" would register a 9.9. This is a very important number for you to remember, for reasons which I will explain later.

Practice Makes Perfect

Talking about levels of arousal can get a little bit abstract after a while. You need to experience them. It's the only way to truly master the system. One of the ways you learn each level is by comparing it to the previous level, or to the following one. "How do I know what a 3 is?" you may ask. It's a little higher than a 2. "How do I know I'm at a 7?" you may wonder. Because you're definitely past a 5 or 6, but you haven't hit an 8. Is this vague? I promise it won't be for very long.

Do note that these numbers are all relative to each other. The important thing is that each level feels slightly different. The only absolute number assignments are 1, which is no arousal, 9.9, which is the point of no return, and 10, which is orgasm. Don't worry if your 4 is another man's 5; there is no such thing as the definitive 3 or the quintessential 6.

All that counts are your own *relative* levels of arousal, and that's all you need to know.

Using numbers to describe your arousal may sound a little silly, but I must ask you to take this number system very, very seriously. I am going to refer to different numbers over and over again throughout the remaining exercises. It's the only way we can communicate clearly enough to guarantee you will learn the program. I don't want to sound like your third-grade teacher, but if you want to master these techniques, you have to practice your scales.

TROUBLESHOOTING TIP: Please don't use these numbers to judge your performance in any way. A "6" is not better than a "3"; a "4" is not worse than a "7." They're just different. There is no good and bad here; there is no right or wrong. You will not be graded and you will not be judged. The only goal is to become more intimate with the subtle changes in your body during your arousal.

What About Your Erection?

You'll notice how I haven't said anything about erections. It is very common for men to equate arousal with erections, but they are *not* one and the same. Arousal is a feeling; it is a subjective sense of excitement that can be experienced throughout the body, though it is typically felt most keenly in the genitals. Erection, on the other hand, refers to hardness of the penis. Erection is a very objective measure of hardness that is a direct reflection of blood flowing into this organ.

A man can feel very aroused—incredibly aroused—yet not be erect. Maybe you've felt this way after a long night of lovemaking when your mind wanted to keep going but your penis called it quits for the night. Or perhaps you've felt this way with a new partner that got you totally excited, but also totally nervous. There are many men who have actually had the experience of being aroused to the point of orgasm without ever being erect.

Maybe you become fully erect at arousal Level 4; maybe you don't get erect until Level 6. Or maybe, like most men, it's different on different days. It doesn't matter right now because we're not going to worry a lot about erections here. Our concern is with your level of arousal. As you have probably learned from your own experience, focusing too intently on your erection has a way of discouraging the process. On the other hand, when you leave it alone, it tends to come home. So don't think about it. Right now, all you need to do is focus on your numbers.

How to Peak

To help you learn your arousal scale I'm going to teach you how to "peak." Reaching a peak means letting your arousal rise to a certain level and then immediately letting it drop back down. For example, you may let your arousal rise to Level 6, then let it fall back down. That's a Level 6 peak. Or you may let your arousal rise to Level 9, then let it fall back down. That's a Level 9 peak. (Remember that we are talking about arousal here, not about erections.) This is different from trying to *maintain* your arousal at a given level, which is known as "plateauing." You will learn how to plateau in the next chapter.

If you find this exercise difficult or frustrating at first, don't sweat it. It takes most men a number of sessions before they really "get it." If you are working with a partner, her input can be a big help since her objective experience of you will be slightly different at each level. Let her know that her observations are welcome.

Exercise 6 takes fifteen or twenty minutes and does not require a partner. Exercise 7 is done with a partner and takes a little bit longer.

Exercise 6: Climbing Everest (solo)

Once again, you need to lie down or sit down and get very comfortable. Put some lubrication on your hand and on your penis. What you are going to do now is start by giving yourself a genital caress the way you learned in Exercise 5. Slowly stroke yourself until you reach what you would consider to be a Level 4 of arousal. That's past the "twinge" stage to the point where you're feeling a low, steady "hum" of arousal. Remember that you are not using a masturbation stroke; you are caressing yourself.

When you get to Level 4, *stop* the stimulation and take a deep breath . . . a really slow deep breath. Check your PC muscle, your hip muscles, and your thigh muscles to make sure they're all really relaxed. Good. Now let your arousal drop back down a couple of levels to a "2." Take your time. You have just had your first "peak" at Level 4.

Once you have dropped to Level 2, start your caress again. This time, see if you can go up to around Level 6. You may need to stroke yourself a little bit faster to get to this slightly higher level. That's fine. When you reach Level 6, stop the stimulation once again. Take a real slow deep breath and let your arousal drop back down a few levels to around a "4." Make sure *all* your muscles are completely relaxed. Great. You have just had a "peak" at Level 6.

You are going to continue this exercise for the next fifteen to twenty minutes. What I want you to do is try to have a peak at Level 4, Level 6, Level 7, Level 8, and Level 9, which is the point just prior to your "point of no return." At each level it's important to stop the stimulation, relax, take a really deep breath, and make sure all of your muscles are relaxed. Always let yourself drop at least one level, preferably two, after each peak.

TROUBLESHOOTING TIP: Try not to bring your arousal up in a spike, like shooting from a Level 3 to a Level 8. You're trying to stretch out your arousal into an extended series of gradually increasing peaks. If you were going to graph your arousal, it would look like a wave, not like a needle.

Don't rush your peaks. Each up and down cycle should take four or five minutes. Stretch them out. Let them build slowly and savor each one. As your peaks get higher and higher, it may become more and more difficult to relax. One way to overcome this is by taking deeper and deeper breaths at each level. If all of this stimulation has made you need to ejaculate, go ahead. Otherwise, you can stop the exercise once you've completed four or five peaks. If you don't get up to Level 8 or Level 9 the first time, that's okay; you will with practice.

Ultimately, you will need to be able to peak at very high levels. This is not hard once you get used to the whole process of peaking. Through repetition you will learn to recognize and become comfortable at your different levels. Believe it or not, it won't be long before you can even differentiate between Levels 8, 8.5, 9, and 9.5. Talk about knowing your own body! This kind of fine sensitivity to your arousal will make multiple orgasm a snap.

Exercise 7: Twin Peaks (with a partner)

Would you like to practice "peaking" with your partner? Here's how. First, you need to lie on your back, close your eyes, and get very comfortable. Your partner is going to begin the exercise by doing a sensate focus genital caress. She should do this nice and slow and focus on her own pleasure. She can use her hands, her mouth, or both. All you should focus on is what you are feeling. This keeps the pressure off both of you.

Once she has started, your partner should say to you, "As I am stroking you, let me know if you reach the point that you think is a Level 4." It doesn't matter how much time it takes. Enjoy her caresses. All you need to do is simply say "4" when you have reached that level. Once you say "4," your partner should stop her caress. Check all of your muscles to make sure they are relaxed. Take a deep breath, and let your arousal drop one or two levels. When your arousal has dropped off sufficiently, let your partner know she can start again. It helps to have agreed on a signal ahead of time, such as a nod, a wink, or a U.S. Air Force thumbs up.

Your partner should start the stimulation again very slowly, in a very focused fashion. She will then say, "Let me know when you reach a Level 6." Enjoy her stimulation until you reach Level 6. Take your time. Then, when you reach Level 6, let her know by saying "6." She should stop the stimulation immediately for at least several seconds. Take a deep breath, make sure all of your muscles are relaxed, and let yourself drop down a couple of levels. Once you have dropped and are ready to start up again, give her the signal to resume.

Continuing in this fashion, try to reach Level 7, Level 8, Level 9, and Level 10, if possible. You may skip a level or two if you wish. Depending on how you are feeling during this exercise you may or may not feel like going all the way to orgasm. If you don't want to, stop the exercise at Level 8, or the level of your choice. The most important thing is not to pressure yourself.

It doesn't matter how high you are able to go right now. All that matters is that you are learning to listen to your body. If you would rather stay at the lower levels for a while, that's fine. If you want to go all the way to Level 10 and have an orgasm, that's great too. It's important to know that it's entirely up to you. You should be able to ask yourself, "What do I want today?" Remember, this is for your pleasure.

If you really take your time you can stretch this exercise out to an hour or so. To make it an even nicer experience for both of you, you may want to begin by giving your partner a genital caress. If she wants to, she could even learn to have her own peaks.

TROUBLESHOOTING TIP: Please note that it is possible to "overpeak." If you hit more than three or four really high peaks in one session, you may find yourself temporarily unable to ejaculate. Don't get scared, and don't call 911. You haven't done anything wrong. I call this phenomenon "penis burnout." It may feel a bit weird, but it does not last. All you need to do is stop the exercise for ten minutes or so and everything should return to normal.

Onward and Upward?

By the time you have completed the exercises in this chapter a few times, you are going to have a much more sophisticated sense of your own arousal. That's really important. If your partner has done these exercises with you, she too will be tuned into your body much more intimately. The more she knows your peaks, the more she can get involved later on, and that makes it more exciting for both of you.

Practice these exercises as much as needed to get truly comfortable with your different levels. Remember that having an orgasm is not your goal. Don't feel like you have to climax every time or *any* time you do the exercise. Feel your way through the exercises each time. If you want to have an orgasm, let it happen. If you don't, don't push it. And don't rush these exercises because you can't wait to get to the finale. You'll only wind up coming back to this chapter later on. You are building your foundation here. It has got to be solid. So take your time; you'll be on the roof soon enough.

Once you've learned your scales you are ready to move on to the next chapter. While some men are eager to continue, some may care to linger. If you're having so much fun you don't want to leave this chapter, feel free to hang out here for a while and refine your sensitivity. After all, you can never be too aware of your own arousal. But do remember that there's a lot more waiting for you when you turn the page.

CHAPTER EIGHT

Orgasm, Ejaculation, and You

Learning to become multiorgasmic is like following a recipe for some very exotic dessert. Before you can make the dessert, all of the ingredients must be available. Chapters 6 and 7 helped us to find and prepare some of the most important "ingredients" for this very special recipe. You've learned about the PC muscle, the key ingredient, and hopefully you are getting yours strong and ready even as we speak. You've learned about sensate focus, demand-free interaction, and the point of no return. You've discovered the many levels of your own arousal and the pleasure of peaking at these levels.

Now we're ready to take out the mixing bowls and start combining some of our ingredients. We also have a few more items to add. I know that you are anxious to get to the crucial exercises just two chapters away, but it won't be long now. Any good chef will tell you that the secret to great cooking is all in the preparation. So relax, take another deep breath, and try to get the most out of these very important exercises.

Peaking with the PC Muscle

Once you have learned how to peak at various levels, you're ready to learn how to use the PC muscle to control those peaks. A strong PC muscle works like a good set of brakes in your car. You can use it to control your arousal the way you use your brakes to control your speed, and you don't even need a learner's permit to start practicing.

But here's the kicker. A strong PC can do a lot more than just control your arousal. It's also the "brake" you will use to hold back your ejaculation while you are having an orgasm.

In the last chapter you learned how to let your arousal drop off by stopping the stimulation at each peak. In the next two exercises, you're going to learn how to get the same results far more effectively by squeezing the PC muscle at those peaks. Learning how to use your brakes during these exercises is a little tricky. That's because there are actually three different ways to squeeze the PC muscle when you are aroused:

• One long hard squeeze, or . . .
• Two medium squeezes, or . . .
• Several quick squeezes in a row

All three methods work, but you'll probably find that one of them usually works best for you. Every man is different, and that means you are going to have to experiment with the different styles of squeezing to find the method that interferes least with your erection while still getting the job done.

Exercise 8 is for those men who will be working alone. Exercise 9 is for men who are working with a partner. These exercises are very important, so take your time.

Exercise 8: King of the Road (solo)

We are going to begin this exercise the same way we started our first peaking exercise in the previous chapter (Exercise 6: "Climbing Everest"). Lie down or sit comfortably and, using plenty of lubrication, begin a genital self-caress. Stroke your penis in a slow, gentle fashion, letting your arousal level gradually rise.

Make your first peak Level 4, a low-level peak. But this time, as you reach Level 4 you are going to *continue* stroking yourself. You are not going to stop the stimulation. Instead, what I want you to do is hit the brakes—that is, give your PC muscle one or two good strong squeezes, or three quick squeezes. Then take a very long and deep breath—lasting several seconds. Once you have done this, stop the stimulation and make sure all of your muscles are relaxed. Now let your arousal drop two levels, to a Level 2.

What you should have noticed is that even though you were still caressing yourself, the PC squeeze stopped your arousal from going any higher. It may have even taken you down one level. To drop two levels, most men need to stop the caress, which is why I ask you to stop the stimulation after your deep breath.

Let's now try for a peak at Level 6. Start your caress and let yourself fully experience the many sensations of your arousal as your level starts to rise. When you reach a Level 6, do not stop your caress. Instead, hit the brakes again, giving your PC one or two firm squeezes, or three quickies. Take a long, deep breath. Now stop your stimulation and let yourself drop to a Level 4.

Try to continue this exercise for the next fifteen or twenty minutes, doing several more peaks. If you can, do a peak at Levels 7, 8, and 9. There are two things you need to know here:

1. The higher you go, the longer and deeper that big breath needs to be.

2. The higher you go, the harder you are going to have to squeeze your PC muscle.

This is especially true at the highest levels. At a Level 9, for example, you are probably going to have to give that PC muscle one or two *really long, really hard squeezes* and you're going to have to take a *really long, really deep breath*. Again, it's just like driving a car. At high speeds, you've got to really slam on those brakes to make a quick stop. So, enjoy the drive, but don't be afraid to really hit your PC brake when the time comes.

Exercise 9: Moonlight Drive
(with a partner)

Peaking with the PC muscle is a great exercise to do with a partner. To begin, lie on your back and get very comfortable. Using plenty of lubrication, your partner should begin a genital caress. She can use manual and/or oral stimulation—whatever *she* prefers. Remember, she is doing the caress for *her* pleasure.

When you reach a Level 4 on your arousal scale, squeeze your PC muscle. Take a long, deep breath. Your PC squeeze should stop your arousal from going any higher, even though your partner has not stopped the stimulation. It could even drop you one level. Your deep breath is a signal to your partner that it is time for her to stop her caress. She should wait until the *end* of your long breath before she actually stops.

Let your arousal drop two full levels. When you are certain you have reached a Level 2, you are ready to continue. Let your partner know that she can start her caress again.

This time, you are going to peak at Level 6. When you reach Level 6, squeeze your PC muscle. Take a long, deep breath. At the end of this breath, your partner should stop all stimulation and let you fall back down to Level 4.

Continue this exercise through Levels 7, 8, and 9. Remember that the higher you go, the harder you have to squeeze that PC muscle. Don't be afraid to really hit those brakes—you can't wear out the pads. That's why you've been working so hard to make the muscle strong. Also, remember that the deep breath you take when you squeeze the PC needs to be longer and deeper at every level.

TROUBLESHOOTING TIP: You're not the only one who might enjoy a few peaks. Whenever you complete a peaking session, ask your partner if she wants one of her own. Even if she doesn't, she'll appreciate your thoughtfulness.

A Position to Envy

Do you think you're ready for a little more excitement? What about your partner? Is she ready too? We haven't talked much about intercourse yet, but I think we're ready to start talking now. Incorporating intercourse into your exercise regimen is the ultimate thrill. The exercises become so exciting and so erotic you'll have a hard time calling them exercises. But, believe it or not, they are still exercises, specifically designed to bring you closer and closer to your goal of multiple orgasm.

If you are getting a fairly strong erection from your partner's caresses, this is a good time to introduce intercourse into the program. Exercise 10 will show you how, but first we need to talk for just a moment about positions. In all of the years my colleagues and I have worked with these techniques, one intercourse position has remained our favorite. It's our experience that this position maximizes the benefits of the techniques you are learning while minimizing effort. I don't want to sound like a mechanical engineer here, but in this position, which you are about to learn, all of the angles are ideal. The motion is ideal and the contact is ideal. Best of all, it *feels* great.

Every couple is different, and it is entirely possible that you may find one or more different positions that work even better for you than the one I recommend. That's fine. I would never want to discourage you from experimenting. Try any position you are interested in. Have fun with it. Play. You may discover your own favorite. But first, let me teach you mine.

The woman should lie on her back and feel very comfortable. She may want a pillow under her buttocks and the small of her back for extra comfort. She raises her legs in the air, spreads them comfortably, and bends her knees. The man should be on his knees, in between the woman's legs. Note that the man is going to use his *knees*, not his arms, to support most of his weight. *It is extremely important that his center of gravity is in his hips.* This minimizes muscle tension in the man's torso, enabling him to fully relax his muscles during the exercise. It is from this position that he penetrates the woman.

Now I know that at first this position may sound a little bit convoluted. After all, we're making love here, not pretzels. But hear me out. You will recall how important it is for you to have your muscles as relaxed as possible during these exercises. In certain intercourse positions, it is simply not possible for these muscles to relax, and that can make learning these techniques far more difficult. The position I have just described also makes it very easy for the man to breathe properly. As I've said before, good breathing technique is extremely important in these exercises. While the position I've described is not the *only* position that works, it is the best one I know . . . particularly when you are learning to become multiorgasmic for the first time. Most men and women tell me that this is the position with which they have their greatest success. They get used to it very quickly, and usually it's the one they come to prefer over all others, regardless of how many they try. So give it a chance. It's hot. Trust me.

If you are not in a committed, monogamous relationship where it has been clearly established that both partners are HIV negative, you must practice safe sex.

Exercise 10: Enter the Dragon
(with a partner)

This exercise begins just like Exercise 9 ("Moonlight Drive"). You are lying on your back and your partner is giving you a sensate focus genital caress. You are going to do a peak at Level 4 and another at Level 6. Each time you will use your PC muscle to put the brakes on your arousal. You will also take a deep, deep breath at these peaks, at which point your partner will stop her caress.

If you have a fairly strong erection by the time you peak at Level 6, you are ready to have intercourse with your partner. (If you don't have a strong erection yet, don't push it. Wait until Level 8 or Level 9.) The first thing you need to do is switch positions. Your partner needs to lie on her back. She should raise her legs in the air, spread them apart sufficiently, and bend her knees comfortably.

You are going to kneel between her legs, with your legs and hips supporting the bulk of your weight. Now you are going to insert your penis and begin slowly, gently thrusting. In this exercise, no speed is too slow. Move your penis in and out of her vagina by rolling or rocking your pelvis. Don't tense your muscles.

This is still a pressure-free sensate focus exercise. Think of yourself as caressing the inside of your partner's vagina with your penis. Focus on the sensations. Stay in the here and now. Don't think about your performance. This is solely for your pleasure. If your mind starts to drift, gently bring yourself back to the pleasurable sensations you are feeling in the moment.

Your partner should be totally focused on her sensations too. If she's really paying attention to what she's feeling, her arousal levels are likely to go up just like yours. The two of you are going to feel really connected here. You're climbing these mountains together.

Peak at Level 7. This may require you to slowly increase the speed of your thrusting. Nothing frantic, just a medium speed. When you reach Level 7, hit the brakes by squeezing your PC (hopefully by now you have discovered the method of squeezing that works best for you). Take a deep, deep breath. Now stop moving. Tell your partner, "That's a 7." This is her cue to stop moving too. Stay inside your partner and wait for your arousal to drop two levels. This should take a few seconds.

Once your arousal has dropped two levels, start thrusting again. This time, you want to peak at Level 8. Try to keep your thrusting at medium speed. You're not in any rush—let your arousal build slowly. When you reach Level 8, squeeze your PC. Take a deep, deep breath. Then stop moving for a few seconds. Tell your partner, "That's an 8." She should stop moving too, if she hasn't already. Stay inside of her and let your arousal drop at least two levels.

You may be ready to stop the exercise by now. Or you may feel like you're just getting started. If you both want to try for a Level 9 peak, go for it. Remember that you are going to have to squeeze that PC *really* hard and take a *really* deep breath when you hit your high peaks. If you want to go all the way to orgasm, that's great too. But feel free to stop at any time. The most important thing is that both of you are enjoying yourselves.

TROUBLESHOOTING TIP: You can learn all you need to know about peaking without having any intercourse. The most important thing right now is that neither you nor your partner are feeling any pressure to perform. If you would prefer to limit your contact to genital caresses, please do. And remember that if you do have intercourse it should be a *pressure-free* interaction. Don't change the intent of the exercises.

CHAPTER NINE

From Peaks to Plateaus

You are now ready to prepare the final ingredient in our recipe for male multiple orgasm: the plateau. A plateau, quite simply, is an extended peak. The peaks you have been creating in the previous chapter last only one or two seconds. Well, imagine taking these short peaks and stretching them out so they last five seconds, ten seconds, or even longer before they drop off. Instead of a quick peak, you now have an exhilarating plateau.

In the following exercises you are going to learn how to stretch your peaks into plateaus lasting anywhere from several seconds to several minutes. This may sound like a long time right now, but once you experience just how wonderful each plateau feels, you're going to wish it lasted even longer. I get excited just thinking about it.

There are four different ways to stretch a peak into a plateau.

- Changing your breathing

- Squeezing your PC muscle

- Changing your motion

- Changing your focus

I'm going to teach you all four of these methods in the following exercises. All four are important, for reasons I will discuss later. What you're really doing in these plateauing exercises is learning how to manipulate and prolong your own arousal using different types of stimulation. You're learning to "play" with your levels—to control them and enjoy them in new and exciting ways. This kind of control is going to pave the way toward your first multiple orgasm.

These techniques are a little bit more tricky than anything you've tried so far, but the rewards are worth the effort. So, assuming you are rested and ready, let's get back to work. Note that Exercise 11 does not require a partner, while Exercise 12 is done with a partner.

Exercise 11: Bronco Buster (solo)

Lie on your back or sit in a chair and get very comfortable. Using plenty of lubrication, begin a genital caress. Start working toward a Level 5 peak. Using the first technique—changing your breathing—you are actually going to stretch that Level 5 peak into a Level 5 plateau.

As you reach Level 5 you want to start thinking about making your first plateau. Pay close attention to your arousal level. You should be getting pretty good at this by now. Can you tell the difference between a "5" and a "5.5"?

Before you reach Level 6, *slow down your breathing*. Don't change anything else. By intentionally slowing your breathing pattern, your arousal level should start to fall. Pay close attention as it starts to dip. Once it drops below Level 5, you want to change your breathing again. This time, you want to *breathe faster*—so you're almost panting. If you are breathing fast enough, your arousal level will rise back to Level 5 or higher.

Just by manipulating your breathing—alternating between slowing it down and speeding it up—

you should be able to hover at Level 5 (plus or minus half a level). A lot of guys call this "riding a 5." See if you can stay there for at least a few seconds.

TROUBLESHOOTING TIP: You don't want to do this particular breathing manipulation too long because you might hyperventilate. Sixty seconds is too long. Ten or fifteen seconds is plenty. You can create longer plateaus with the other three techniques.

Take a rest, letting your arousal drop one or two levels. Then begin stroking yourself again so your arousal starts to climb. This time, let's try to plateau at Level 6 using the second technique: squeezing the PC muscle.

As you reach Level 6 you want to be thinking about your plateau. Don't stop your caress. Let your arousal continue to rise. But by the time you reach Level 6.5, you need to take action. It's simple: give your PC a couple of squeezes. That's all. Don't change anything else; this time it is only the PC you're going to work with.

Squeezing the PC should stop your arousal from climbing any higher, and could bring you down half a level or more. Continue your caress with the same intensity and let your level rise again. Every time you pass Level 6 use the PC to bring you back down. Try to "ride" that Level 6 for at least ten or fifteen seconds. Yeehaa! You've created a plateau with the PC muscle.

Now let's try the third technique: changing your motion. This time, you are going to stretch your peak into a plateau by changing the speed at which you stroke your penis. Begin as though you were going to peak at Level 7. Once you have passed Level 7, slow your motion down. The shift should lower your arousal almost immediately. Let yourself dip below a "7." Now speed up your motion to rise back up.

Whenever you want to raise your level, speed up your stroke. Whenever you want to drop it, slow down. It's that simple. Try to maintain your Level 7 plateau for at least a few seconds. Have a good ride.

The fourth way to stretch a peak into a plateau is to change the focus. In this exercise, changing the focus means changing the area of your genitals that you are stimulating (it will have a different meaning in other exercises). Let's say you've been caressing the head of your penis. To change the focus, you'd stop touching the head and start caressing the testicle or the shaft. Sound simple? Good. Let's try it.

This time, let's shoot for Level 8. Caress yourself as though you were going to peak at Level 8, but when you hit your "8," don't stop. Somewhere between "8" and "8.5" you want to change the focus of your caress. Your arousal should start to drop. As your arousal dips below Level 8, shift back to the area you were touching before or intensify the pressure of your touch. This should bring you back up. If you get too high, shift again. Use this technique to extend your Level 8 peak into a ten- or fifteen-second plateau.

Congratulations cowboy! You're a full-fledged bronco buster now.

TROUBLESHOOTING TIP: The key to mastering the plateau is learning to stay relaxed while you continue to stimulate yourself. This gets easier to do once you trust that the four different techniques you've just learned really work. With some practice, you can learn to ride at really intense levels, such as Level 9 or even Level 9.5.

You can also learn how to plateau with your partner. Extending your arousal extends your partner's pleasure too, making this exercise a favorite among women. Some men find it easier to learn plateauing techniques with a partner whereas others find it easier to work alone. Try it both ways, if you like, and see what's best for you.

Exercise 12: Endless Summer
(with a partner)

Once again, you need to lie on your back and get comfortable. Your partner is going to begin a sensate focus genital caress. This is a demand-free exercise. You should both be focusing on the sensations—nothing more.

Your first plateau is going to be at Level 4, and you are going to create it by controlling your breathing. As you reach Level 4, start breathing more slowly and deeply. Your arousal should start to drop, even though your partner is continuing her caress. When you dip to a "3.5" start breathing faster, as though you were panting. Your level should rise. Slow down your breathing again once you pass Level 4.

By alternating between slow breathing and panting, you should be able to maintain your plateau at Level 4 for ten or fifteen seconds. It's like catching a wave and riding it. Just remember that you don't want to manipulate your breathing for very long because you run the risk of hyperventilating.

Try your next plateau at Level 6. This time, you're going to use your PC muscle to help you ride the wave.

Your partner is continuing her caress. Your arousal level is rising. When you reach a point just beyond Level 6, give your PC muscle a couple of squeezes. Your level should stop rising—it could even drop slightly.

Your partner is still continuing her caress. Focus on her stimulation. Every time your level hits "6.5," squeeze that muscle. Try to hold this plateau for at least fifteen seconds. Now let's try a plateau at Level 7 with the third technique: changing your motion. In the last exercise, you changed your hand motion. But you're working with a partner now. So in this exercise, you're going to change the motion of your pelvis.

As your partner caresses you, try responding with some gentle thrusts and rolls of your pelvis. Nothing too quick or abrupt, and nothing too stiff. Just nice, easy thrusts and rolls. Let your arousal rise.

Once you pass Level 7, slow down or stop your pelvic motion. Your level should start to drop, even though your partner is continuing her caress. If you dip below "7," speed up your movements. Your level should start to rise again. It's that simple. Using this technique, try to ride Level 7 for at least fifteen seconds.

Now let's try the fourth technique—switching the focus—to create a plateau at Level 8.

In chapter 6 you learned how to focus all of your attention on the areas that you or your partner were touching at that very moment. But it is also possible to intentionally shift your focus to an area that is *not* being touched at that moment. This is different from changing the area where you are being touched, as you did in the previous exercise. This time, you are only making a *mental* shift in your focus.

Let's say that your partner has been focusing her caress on the head of your penis. Your attention has been focused there too. By now, that area is feeling extremely sensitive and you are very aroused. As you pass Level 8, try shifting your mental focus to an area she is not stimulating as intensely. Focus on the shaft of your penis, for example. Or focus on the feeling of her body lying across yours. Your level should start to drop.

If your level dips below "8," shift your focus back to the area on which your partner is concentrating. Your level should start to rise again. That's all there is to it. If you want to go higher, focus on the area being stimulated. If you want to go lower, focus on an area not being stimulated so intensely.

This is not the same as thinking about baseball or your old Aunt Irma. You are not trying to mentally leave the room. You are staying very connected to your body and very connected to your partner. You are only changing the point of connection.

Using this fourth technique, you should be able to maintain a plateau at Level 8 for at least fifteen seconds, if not more.

TROUBLESHOOTING TIP: You don't *have* to work in any particular order and you don't *have* to work at any particular level. I just find that it tends to be easier when you work from low to high. I also don't recommend doing more than four plateaus in any one session. Save something for next time.

Student Driver on Board

You have now learned four different ways to create a plateau. Some may appeal to you more than others, or work more effectively than others, but the truth is, the best way to create long, fabulous plateaus is to use these four techniques *all together*.

Now that may sound a bit mind boggling. At this point, you've barely mastered each one individually. But it's a lot like learning to drive a car. Remember how you felt when you got behind the wheel for the first time? There you were, staring down at the clutch, the stick, the brakes, the gas, and the turn signals, thinking, "How am I ever going to learn to do all of these things at the same time?" But you did, didn't you?

When you learned to drive a car, you didn't start by doing everything at once. You added things in, one or two at a time. Well, that's what you're going to do in these plateauing exercises. So spend some time with these exercises. When you get comfortable with one plateauing technique, try to add a second, and then a third. Before you know it, working simultaneously with all four methods will be almost automatic.

Don't worry if you're not a quick study. You don't *have* to work with all four techniques simultaneously to have great plateaus. It's just easier when you're using all four together. That's probably hard to imagine right now, but you'll understand once you've had a little practice.

Feel Like Makin' Love?

It's nice to be beside your partner when you're learning how to create plateaus for the first time. But once you've started getting comfortable with your newest techniques, it might be even nicer to be *inside* her.

There's something about being inside a woman that gives most men extra incentive to stretch out those plateaus. Your partner is going to be just as into these exercises as you are; she may even be doing a little plateauing of her own. A lot of women who are multiorgasmic are actually plateauing at Level 9.9. Their arousal is up so high for so long that they just start crossing over to Level 10 over and over, having orgasm after orgasm. You're going to learn a different method—something that works better for men—but I thought you'd appreciate knowing this little piece of multiple orgasm trivia.

If you can have intercourse without putting any pressure on yourself or on your partner, try having a few plateaus inside your partner. Experiment with maintaining different levels of arousal during intercourse. The four techniques you will be using are the same: changing your breathing, squeezing your PC muscle, changing your motion, and changing your focus. Be adventurous. Party. Just don't forget that you both have jobs to go to on Monday morning.

Please do remember that you don't have to have intercourse in any of these exercises to make them wonderful and special. If you're still most comfortable with the genital caress, stay with it for now. There will be plenty of opportunities for intercourse later on, once you have solidified your new skills. The most important thing right now is to just keep practicing, and practicing, and practicing. . . .

CHAPTER TEN

Your First Multiple Orgasm

Allison and Daniel, who you read about in the beginning of this book, are once again making love on a Sunday morning. They are the same two people they were a month ago, but they don't feel like the same two people.

Their lovemaking started when Daniel walked out of the shower and was greeted by Allison, who was wearing nothing but a large blue and white striped bath towel. When she wrapped the towel around the two of them, Daniel responded immediately.

Right now they are on top of their queen-size bed where they have been making love for the last ten minutes. They are both totally turned on, and Daniel feels he is ready to have an orgasm, but Daniel knows that Allison needs another five minutes of intercourse before she can climax. *No problem.*

What was once a source of incredible stress for Daniel and disappointment for Allison is no longer. Daniel knows that this time he can have a powerful orgasm without disturbing the erotic connection. Allison, who knows that Daniel's orgasm does not signal the end of their lovemaking, becomes even more excited. It's thrilling for her to be with Daniel, knowing that he can climax and still keep going.

After his first orgasm, Daniel is able to maintain his erection and continue thrusting until Allison also reaches orgasm. Allison is so excited by Daniel that she actually reaches her climax much sooner than he had anticipated.

Daniel feels that he could keep going for another twenty minutes, but the chime of the grandfather clock in the hall reminds him that they are supposed to meet friends for brunch, and that they had better start moving in that direction. At this point, Daniel decides to have his second orgasm. This time, he will ejaculate.

Until recently, Daniel, like you, knew only one type of orgasm: a single orgasm accompanied by simultaneous ejaculation. Not anymore. Today, he understands that:

• Orgasm and ejaculation do not have to occur together; they are two distinct phenomena that can be experienced as separate pleasures.

• A nonejaculatory orgasm feels as good, if not better, than a conventional orgasm.

• Having a nonejaculatory orgasm enables you to maintain an erection and continue intercourse.

• It is possible to have a second orgasm soon after your first orgasm. It is even possible to have a third or fourth orgasm, whether or not you ejaculate with any or all of your orgasms. Daniel has learned all of this through his own experience. Now it is time for you to learn.

You are about to have your first multiple orgasm. Prepare yourself—life may never be quite the same again. You have reached this point because you have worked hard. You have turned weak muscle into steel, mastered the most subtle nuances of your own physiology, ascended difficult peaks, and traversed many daunting plateaus. You may even have slain a dragon or two along the way.

You have met all the challenges, and probably had quite a bit of fun doing so. It's time to rid both you and your damsel of your distress.

In this chapter you will learn the techniques that will transform you from a mild-mannered orgasmic man into a multiorgasmic superhero. If you have followed my instructions carefully and done your homework thoroughly, the transformation will not be difficult. You will not need a phone booth. You will not need tights and a cape. You will not need to hide your identity from your loved ones. In this legion of superheroes, enthusiasm and a bit of hard work are the only requirements for admission.

Two Ways to the Top

As you will soon see, the key to separating orgasm from ejaculation lies in the proper use of a well-developed PC muscle. If you are not yet confident in the power of your PC, now is the time to go back to the earlier exercises and build the necessary strength. You'll get to the good stuff soon enough, and your patience and efforts will be rewarded in extraordinary ways. If, on the other hand, your PC has done its job to your satisfaction in all of the previous exercises, you are probably ready to take the final steps.

There are actually many paths to achieving male multiple orgasm. In this chapter, you're going to learn two of them. These choices have not been made arbitrarily. The two methods in this chapter are the two methods in which I have the most confidence. They are the methods my colleagues and I have worked with the most and like the most.

The first method you are going to learn is what we call the "one-shot" technique. It is a shortcut of sorts that was developed by my colleague and mentor Dr. Michael Riskin. Dr. Riskin calls it a one-shot technique because he can usually teach the technique in only one office session (assuming you've done all of the preparatory work presented in the preceding chapters). You walk into the office a man, and you walk out a multiorgasmic man. Amazing.

The second method is the one I teach most often in private practice with my clients. I'm a bit more conservative than some of my colleagues, and this method takes a little bit longer to learn, whether you are learning at home or at my office. But the results are always impressive.

At the clinic, we like to tease each other about whose techniques are best. It certainly makes for interesting conversation at the water cooler, but we all know that our opinions are only our opinions. The truth is, every client has his own preferences, and there is no way to predict yours. As I've said before, every man is slightly different, and what works best or feels best for one does not work as well or feel as good for the next. We have all seen the effectiveness of both methods and we know they're both good. In this chapter, you'll have the opportunity to experiment with both and decide for yourself.

Fairy Tales Can Come True (Or, The Tortoise and the Hare Revisited)

Dr. Riskin's one-shot technique is the fastest way I know for a man to reach his first multiple orgasm. It is also easier to learn than the second method. When it works, it's amazing. But please take note: *The one-shot technique does not work for every man.* It is a shortcut, and shortcuts do not always work. The second method in this chapter is far more thorough and far more foolproof. It takes a little more time to learn, but the payoff awaits.

If this one-shot method does not work for you, you have absolutely no reason to get discouraged. It does not mean that there is something wrong with your equipment and it does not mean that you will never have a multiple orgasm. All it means is that you spent a few minutes trying something new, and it didn't work. You will learn the one-shot method first because it does save time.

If the one-shot technique does not work for you, do not stop. Do not pass GO. Do not skip a turn. Do not pack your bags and head for Fiji. Instead, please go immediately to the second set of exercises in this chapter. These more comprehensive techniques are not harder to learn. There are more steps in the process, but it is not a difficult process if you follow my instructions. Yes, it may take you a bit longer before you have your first multiple orgasm, but you *will* have it. Plus, you will also have learned a valuable lesson about the benefits of patience and commitment. Then someday, years from now, when you are sitting with your great-grandchildren reading "The Tortoise and the Hare," you'll remember these moments, and tell the story with much greater conviction.

No Cheating, Please

Before we get started, let me stress one last time that the techniques presented in this chapter require a powerful PC muscle that is under your control. This is especially true for the one-shot technique. You also need to be very confident in your ability to peak and/or plateau at very high arousal levels.

I can appreciate the fact that you want to get to the good stuff, and I applaud your enthusiasm. It must be hard *not* to rush when nirvana awaits, but this is another instance in which rushing can ruin sex.

My grandfather used to say, "It's hard to reach nirvana if the tires on the bus don't have enough air." (I guess you can understand why he and my grandmother got along so well.) Please take a moment right now to "check your tires." Please examine how diligent you have been following the exercise regimen until this point. Be honest with yourself. If you are the least bit unsure about how thorough you've been, now is the time to go back to the earlier exercises and really give it your all.

There is only one shortcut in this book, and that's the one you're about to learn. If you have tried to cut corners with any of the previous exercises, you are going to be very frustrated and disappointed when you attempt the exercises in this chapter. Achieving male multiple orgasm is easy if you do the work, but if you don't do the work, it usually doesn't happen.

The Shot Heard Round the World

Exercises 13 and 14 were developed by Dr. Michael Riskin through his work with hundreds of men at the Riskin-Banker Psychotherapy Center. He has spent many years refining and perfecting his techniques, and I am happy to be able to present them here. Even if this method doesn't work for you, it's fun to try. So go for it. Exercise 13 is done with a partner and Exercise 14 is done without a partner.

Exercise 13: Doc Riskin's Magic Motion (with a partner)

This exercise begins with the man lying on his back. Your partner begins by giving you a genital caress with her hands and/or mouth. Let your arousal build. The first thing you are going to do is peak at Level 4. When you reach Level 4, let your partner know. She should stop the stimulation and let you drop a couple of levels. Use your PC to help control the situation.

Ask your partner to resume the stimulation. When you reach Level 5, let her know. She should stop again and let you drop a couple of levels. Use your PC if you need to. Now start again and do a peak to Level 6. It should take between three and five minutes to complete each peak. If you want to take more time, stretch your peaks into plateaus using the techniques we practiced in the previous chapter.

At this point you are going to get into the position we have been using for intercourse. You should be feeling pretty aroused right now, and you probably have at least a partial erection if not a full erection.

Insert your penis into your partner and begin slowly thrusting. You should be taking slow, focused, deep breaths the entire time. Focus on what you are feeling. Focus on every thrust. Your partner should also be focusing on the thrusts and focusing on her feelings.

TROUBLESHOOTING TIP: The two of you are in this together. If your partner is counting the cracks in the ceiling, it defeats the whole purpose of these techniques. Only practice the partner exercises when both of you are really into it. If you want to practice and she doesn't, fly solo.

Peak up to Level 7. When you reach Level 7, either slow down or stop thrusting until your arousal drops a couple of levels. Stay in the moment. Now resume or accelerate your thrusting and peak up to Level 8. Let your arousal drop a couple of levels once again. Next, peak up to Level 9. Then drop down yet again. You may prefer to take more time by stretching these peaks into longer plateaus.

Now here's the tricky part. This time you are going to resume thrusting past Level 9, all the way to your point of inevitability. (Remember that's the psychological point where it becomes clear to you that ejaculation is going to happen, no matter what.) *As soon as you hit your point of no return, squeeze your PC muscle as hard as you can for ten seconds and open your eyes. Take a really deep breath. Now keep thrusting! Don't stop!*

TROUBLESHOOTING TIP: Most people instinctively close their eyes as they approach orgasm. To make this technique work, you *must* open your eyes during the PC squeeze. I don't know why. All I know is that it doesn't work if you keep your eyes closed. Keeping the eyes open is the part of this technique that men are most likely to forget.

If you can do all of these things simultaneously, your body is going to go into orgasm at this very moment. Your heart will pound, you'll sweat, and your muscles will contract. All of the sensations of at least a partial, if not a full, orgasm will be there. *But you will not ejaculate.* Your PC has stopped your ejaculation while still allowing your body to go into orgasm.

Once you've experienced this partial or full orgasm you need to slow down for a while. Relax for a few seconds—you've earned it. You can continue thrusting, but it shouldn't be vigorous.

Instead, begin some real slow, easy thrusting accompanied by some slow breathing.

Right now you're probably marveling at the fact that you've just had an orgasm and you're still thrusting. Your partner is probably marveling at it too. Pat yourself on the back. Pat each other on the back. Pat each other anywhere you want. But remember, we're not done yet. One down, one to go.

Once you are in control of your breathing again, it's time to start back toward the top. Slowly increase the speed of your thrusting. Keep your focus. Let your arousal level rise once more. If you want to do more peaks or plateaus, go ahead. But at this point you may prefer to just let yourself go straight to the top. (Please note that at this point you simply are learning to have two orgasms in a single session of intercourse. In chapter 11 we will talk more about lengthening the amount of time between orgasms, having more than two orgasms, etc.)

When you feel your orgasm coming on once again, don't try to manipulate it. Don't try to stop your ejaculation this time. You've done enough work for one day. Focus fully on the sensations of your arousal, and let yourself have a second climax—ejaculation and all.

Now you really need to congratulate yourself and each other. *You have just had your first multiple orgasm.*

I suspect that one of the reasons why the one-shot method doesn't work for every man is because, as you may have already discovered, it is hard to do. There are so many things to coordinate, particularly at the point where you have to squeeze your

PC, take a deep breath, open your eyes, and keep thrusting—all at the same time. That's harder than learning to play the piano.

The good news is that your partner can be extremely helpful here. If she is keeping pace with you, her actions can reinforce your actions. It helps a lot if she takes a deep breath when you take a deep breath. It helps if she keeps moving as a reminder for you to keep moving. And if she opens her eyes and sees that you haven't opened yours, she can tell you.

One and a Half Orgasms Are Better Than One

Some men have two full orgasms the first time they try the one-shot technique. Some men cannot work with this method at all. But most men fall somewhere in between. For these men, the first few attempts at mastering the one-shot technique yield some unusual results.

Whether you are practicing the one-shot technique or the second, more conservative method, which will be presented shortly, you are likely to experience any number of new and/or unusual sensations before you have your first true multiple orgasm. For example:

- You may feel like you missed an orgasm.

- You may have a partial orgasm that isn't terribly impressive.

- You may have a partial ejaculation without an orgasm after you have your first orgasm.

All of these responses are completely normal. There is absolutely nothing to worry about. In fact, these seemingly strange physiological experiences are all clear signs that you are on your way to having your first full multiple orgasm. Did you hear that? These are *good* signs, not bad signs. *Most* men who are learning to become multiorgasmic have at least one of these unusual responses before their techniques really "click." It's all part of the process. If you aren't expecting it, it can be kind of scary. But if you are expecting it, it's positive reinforcement.

So put away your worry beads, cancel your appointment with the urologist, and get back to work. Your first *full* multiple orgasm awaits . . . and it won't be long now.

Last-Minute Jitters Before the Big Debut?

Having your first multiple orgasm is a very big deal. Some men want to share every moment of it with their partners whereas other men get a little nervous and prefer to gain some mastery over these techniques before they host their first coming-out party. Like most of the exercises in this book, the one-shot method can be learned with or without a partner. It's really up to you and your partner to decide whether or not your first multiple orgasm will be a private event or a semiprivate event (though I discourage you from trying to sell the rights to pay-per-view).

If you are feeling a bit nervous about having your first multiple orgasm, Exercise 14 will teach you how to master the one-shot technique without a partner. Once you've had a few multiple orgasms on your own and you're feeling more confident, you can then return with your partner to Exercise 13.

Even if you have your first multiple orgasm with your partner, you may want to practice the one-shot technique on your own at some point. If this is the case, Exercise 14 is the exercise for you. Many men like to practice without a partner and some wouldn't have it any other way. This doesn't mean they don't love their partners. It just means they're driven to excel. One client recently told me, "Practicing on my own was an essential part of learning the fine points of my personal response. I have incredible control now. I think it would have been much harder to develop that if I was always doing this with my partner." As always, your approach to learning these techniques is a choice for you and your partner to make. There is no right or wrong way.

Exercise 14: One-Man Mission to Mars (solo)

This exercise begins like a peaking exercise. Using plenty of lubrication, begin stroking your penis. Feel your arousal level start to rise. The first thing you want to do is peak at Level 4 using your PC muscle (the way you did in Exercises 4 and 5). After you have dropped a couple of levels, intensify your stimulation and do a peak at Level 6. Once again, use your PC muscle to control your peak. Next, peak at Level 8. Then at Level 9. Take your

time. These first four peaks should take at least fifteen or twenty minutes to complete. (If you want
to take even more time, try to plateau at each of
these levels.)

What you are going to do now is really push
this peaking exercise. Intensify your stimulation
once again and peak to Level 9.5. Use your PC muscle to stop your arousal from increasing. You need
to be really in control of your body to do this.
You're getting very close to the top now and the
temptation to let yourself go and have an orgasm is
enormous. Hang in there if you can. It won't be long
now.

Your final peak is going to be *at* the point of
inevitability—your psychological point of no return
where ejaculation feels imminent. Talk about danc-
ing on the volcano. This is the toughest peak you'll
ever climb.

You have to be totally tuned in to your body
right now. You're going to be stroking your penis
intensely, heading right toward ejaculation. But the
moment you reach your point of inevitability—not
one second later, but at that very moment—you
want to slam on the PC muscle. *Keep stroking* your
penis just as fast as you've been stroking up to this
point. *Take a really deep breath.* Now *open your eyes*
and keep them open. Hold your PC muscle as tight
as you can for about *ten seconds.*

Whew ... I get exhausted just describing it. If
you can do all of these things at your point of
inevitability, what will happen here is that your
body will go into orgasm. But if you've squeezed
hard enough and long enough with your PC, *you
will not ejaculate.*

TROUBLESHOOTING TIP: It may sound silly, but you *must* open your eyes the moment you start your PC squeeze to make this technique work. Besides, this is an event you don't want to miss.

Take a deep breath again. Slow down the stimulation and let your arousal dip down to Level 8 or Level 7. You're going to be very tired at this point, and probably pretty sweaty. But you're not far from having your first multiple orgasm.

Once you've "rested" for a moment, intensify your stimulation once again. Let your arousal level rise. But this time, you don't want to get in the way. You don't want to squeeze your PC muscle and you don't want to slow your motion. All you want to do is let yourself have a full orgasm, complete with ejaculation. And that, my friend, is a multiple orgasm.

I have said it before but I need to say it again. The first few times you try an exercise like this you may experience any number of unusual sensations, such as a partial orgasm or a "skipped" orgasm. These things may not feel very normal but they all *are* very normal, and there is no reason to be concerned. Your body is learning something new, and these are all encouraging signs of your development. So don't worry . . . be happy.

One other thing. Please remember that this technique does not work for every man. It is difficult to coordinate so many important actions at the exact point of inevitability, but failure to do so may leave you with less than impressive results. Do not despair. It's full speed ahead, on to the second method! As I said earlier, the second method is a bit more work, but it is also far more foolproof.

Three Steps to Higher Consciousness

When I teach men how to have multiple orgasms, I tend to use a more conservative approach than the one-shot method. Because I am a woman, I don't like to make any assumptions about what the average man can or cannot do with his equipment. The conservative approach takes into account a wide range of differences among men, and that makes me feel more confident that it will work for you, the reader. If I were a music teacher, I would probably start all of my students with classical music theory and technique. It might not be as much fun in the beginning, but it's a solid foundation you can work from forever.

At the clinic, it usually takes three sessions to learn this longer method. I guess you could call it a "three-shot technique," or a "three-step program." In the first session, you learn the finer points of ejaculation awareness using two exercises as a learning aid. In the second session, I introduce the exercises that result in multiple orgasm. In the third session, we work on timing and practice. We're going to do the same thing here, but instead of having three sessions in the office, you will learn all three steps in the comfort of your own home. In this chapter, the first two steps are presented. The third step is in chapter 11.

Step 1: An Ejaculation Education

How much do you know right now about your own ejaculation? Did you know, for example, that ejaculation actually occurs in two phases: emission and expulsion? If you did, you get an A in biology. If you didn't, it's time to learn.

In the emission phase of your ejaculation, semen starts to move through the vas deferens as muscles near the prostate gland begin to spasm. The semen then collects in the urethral bulb at the base of the penis. In the second phase of your ejaculation—the expulsion phase—the PC muscle starts to contract, forcing the semen up through the urethra and out of the penis.

That's all very interesting . . . but what did I just say? I'm not so sure myself. I think what we need here is a slightly less academic approach. Let's start by identifying all of the players in this little drama. The vas deferens are a bunch of ducts that carry semen from the testicles to the penis—a sort of semen subway. The prostate gland sits just behind the penis at the tip of the bladder. The prostate is also a source of semen, and if you're one of the lucky ones, that's all you'll ever need to know about the prostate. The urethra, an extension of the bladder, is that little tube that runs up through the center of the penis. It carries both urine and semen out into the fresh air. Is that a little clearer? To make it clearer still, you may want to take a look at the diagram in Appendix 2.

Now let's return to those two phases. In a nutshell, here's what's happening. In the emission phase, semen from the testicles and prostate takes a little subway ride to the base of the penis, prodded along by the contractions of muscles near the prostate gland. In the expulsion phase, your old friend the PC muscle picks up the ball and pushes the semen up through the penis and out into the world. Phase 1: The cannon is loaded. Phase 2: The cannon is fired. It's that simple.

The entire ejaculation process—emission and expulsion—takes about two seconds. Think about that for a moment. Think of all the amazing things you've done for that two-second payoff. Think of the poetry you've written, the florists you've supported, the stories you've woven. . . . Nature is truly amazing.

Why do you need to know all of this? Not so that you will feel foolish. Honest. It is very important for you to have a full understanding of your own ejaculation process, including the timing, if you are going to be a master of your own body. For most men, the contraction of the PC during expulsion is an involuntary process. Once you take control of your PC muscle, however, you can voluntarily delay or prevent ejaculation. Yet your body still experiences the full sensation of orgasm, complete with rapid heart rate, muscle contractions, and the intense sensation of release.

Understanding the difference between emission and expulsion helps you learn to actually *feel* these two distinct phases of ejaculation as they are happening to you. Most men are very aware of the expulsion phase, but they have little sense of what's happening prior to that. But if you want to get the timing right in the last and most important set of exercises in this book, you're going to need a bit more ejaculation awareness than the average guy. That's why I always teach my clients the following exercise.

Exercise 15: Texas Two-Step
(with a partner)

Lie on your back and ask your partner to begin a genital caress. Do a series of low-level peaks—like a Level 4, a Level 5, and a Level 6. Give your partner lots of feedback so she knows when to back off and when to intensify her caress. Once you have completed these peaks, switch positions.

Your partner should now be lying on her back with her legs in the air, slightly bent. You are going to insert your penis and start some slow, comfortable thrusting. Taking plenty of time, peak up to Level 7, then back off. Next, peak up to Level 8, then back off. Now peak up to Level 9, then back off.

Finally, thrust all the way up to your point of inevitability. But this time, the moment you reach the point of inevitability, both you *and* your partner should *stop thrusting*. Keep taking deep breaths, open your eyes, focus all of your attention on your genitals, and try to *feel* the semen moving from your testicles, to the base of your penis, and up through the urethra.

Could you feel the semen collecting? Did you feel your PC spasm? If you stopped thrusting in time, your two-second ejaculation probably felt as if it took five to ten seconds.

*   *   *

Most men thrust all the way through orgasm when they are having intercourse. It would never occur to the average man that there could be benefits to stopping. That should make this exercise a novel experience for most of you. Many men tell me this exercise gives them the feeling that they are in an altered state of consciousness. It is very normal to feel a little bit spacy, transcendent, or out of your body.

Your partner's feedback can also be very helpful here. If she felt that your ejaculation had more throbs than usual, or that it went on for a few more seconds than usual, ask her to let you know. What did it feel like to her? For most women, this exercise is a real turn-on.

Once you have successfully completed this exercise, you're going to have a very different understanding of your own ejaculation. The first thing you're going to notice is how much time you have between your perceived point of no return and the actual expulsion stage of your ejaculation. Time to make a few phone calls, pay a few bills . . . well . . . more time than you thought. You should also see that you have lots of time to squeeze your PC muscle and pull back from the brink of ejaculation if you choose to. Your ejaculation may *feel* inevitable once you've reached your point of no return, but you actually would have plenty of time to stop it if you wanted.

This new understanding of your ejaculation process should give you more confidence in your ability to control your physiology, even at very intense levels of arousal. Hopefully, this confidence will minimize any tendency to panic during Step 2. But before we get to that, here's an exercise to help you learn ejaculation awareness without the help of a partner.

Exercise 16: The Longest Yard (solo)

Lie down on your back and get very comfortable (or sit in a comfortable chair). This exercise begins like a peaking exercise. Using plenty of lubrication, begin stroking your penis and experiencing your arousal. Peak at Level 4, then let your arousal drop two levels. Now peak at Level 6, then let your arousal drop off. Take plenty of time. Each peak should take at least three minutes. Resume your stroking and peak at Level 8. Once again, allow your arousal to drop off two levels before intensifying the stimulation. Peak at Level 9. Remember to breathe deeply as you let your arousal drop off once more.

Intensify your stimulation and let your arousal rise all the way to your point of inevitability. *Now stop stroking.* Open your eyes and focus all of your attention on your genitals. Breathe deeply and regularly as you begin to ejaculate. Can you feel the semen collecting at the base of your penis? Can you feel it when the PC muscle begins to spasm? Can you feel the semen as it moves up through the penis? If you stopped stroking at the right time, your two-second ejaculation should *feel* as though it lasted at least five or six seconds, if not longer. As I mentioned in the previous exercise, feelings of spaciness or altered consciousness are very common when practicing this technique.

STEP 2: THE KEYS TO THE KINGDOM

Now that you have a little bit of ejaculation awareness under your belt, so to speak, you are ready for the coup de grace. The following two exercises are my absolute favorite ways to teach men how to have multiple orgasms. If you found the one-shot technique to be awkward, problematic, or less than satisfactory in any way—as some men do—these are the exercises for you. I love these exercises and the way that my clients respond to them. Frankly, I've never met a man who didn't share my enthusiasm once he followed all of my instructions and suggestions.

Exercise 17 is for a couple to do together, and Exercise 18 is for the man who would prefer to learn on his own. You have worked long and hard to get to this point. Today, a whole new world awaits. Your deepest fantasies are about to come true. It's time for the big payoff. The keys to the kingdom will soon be yours. Are there any cliches I've left out? I don't think so. It's time for us to get to work.

Exercise 17: The Big Takeoff
(with a partner)

You are going to need a full hour to do this exercise. If there's one exercise you don't want to rush, believe me, it's this one. The exercise begins with the man lying on his back, receiving a sensate focus genital caress from his partner. Focus on how good your partner's caress feels as your arousal level begins to rise. Your partner should be focused on touching you, and how sensual that feels to her.

The first thing you are going to do is peak at Level 4, then let your arousal drop two levels. Take your time; both of you should be enjoying all the sensations. Next, do a peak at Level 5 and drop back down. Follow this with a peak at Level 6. Each peak should take at least three or four minutes. Once you have dropped down a bit from Level 6, you are ready to switch positions.

Your partner should lie on her back with her legs up and her knees bent. You want to be on your knees, with most of your weight being supported by your legs. You are going to do a series of peaks while having intercourse with your partner, *but these peaks are going to be very different* from any peaks you've done before. From this point forward you're going to be doing a series of really fast, intense peaks using vigorous thrusting. And you're going to be doing a lot of concentrated, powerful squeezing with your PC muscle. You're not going to take a lot of time in between peaks here. This is a sprinting exercise, and it's going to be very intense.

Begin by inserting your penis into your partner and gently thrusting. Pick up speed quickly. Now thrust as hard as you can until your arousal hits Level 8. *Stop thrusting and squeeze your PC muscle really hard. Your partner should stop thrusting too. Take a deep breath and open your eyes.* Let your arousal drop a level.

===

TROUBLESHOOTING TIP: This exercise works best when your partner's experience mirrors yours. This does not require any acting skills. This exercise should be just as intense for her as it is for you, and it is important that she feels free to express that. There is only one catch. No matter how much she wants to keep going, *the moment you stop thrusting, she must stop moving too.*

===

Once you've dropped a level, start doing some relaxed, easy thrusting. Try to change the angle of entry slightly so that your penis is pointing up higher into your partner. As soon as you've mobilized enough energy, start thrusting as fast and hard as you can. When you reach Level 8.5, *stop thrusting and squeeze your PC muscle really hard.* Your partner should stop thrusting too. *Take a deep breath and open your eyes.* Let yourself drop a level.

As soon as you have your energy back, you want to take off again for another sprint up the hill. Try to point your penis even higher this time. Thrust as hard and as fast as you can all the way to Level 9. Then *stop thrusting and squeeze your PC as hard as you can.* Your partner should stop too. *Take a deep breath and open your eyes.* Back off a level.

This is where it's going to start getting really interesting. Once again, you want to slightly increase your "angle of attack." By the time this exercise is done, your penis is going to be entering your partner at almost a *ninety-degree* angle! Are you ready? This time, you're going to thrust your way to *Level 9.5* before you stop and squeeze your PC. Remember that the higher your arousal level, the harder you have to squeeze and the deeper you need to breathe.

Drop a level and collect your strength. Ready? This time, you're aiming for *Level 9.75!* Point your penis even higher than the last time. Now thrust as fast as you can until you hit your peak. Then stop thrusting, squeeze your PC as hard as you can, take a deep, deep breath, and open your eyes. Your partner should stop moving *the moment* you stop. Any extra motion right now could cause you to ejaculate before you want to.

Your final peak is going to be at Level 9.9 . . . your point of inevitability. This is the big one. Don't panic. Remember how much time you have between the point of inevitability and the expulsion phase of your ejaculation. Your penis should now be pointed as high as it can go. Start your sprint. Thrust as hard and as fast as you can all the way up to your point of inevitability. *Now stop thrusting! Slam on your PC muscle*—give it everything you've got. *Take a huge breath. Open your eyes.* Now try to hold that PC squeeze for at least five to ten seconds.

Right now, your body should be going into orgasm. Your heart is pounding, your muscles are contracting, and you're probably sweating—*but you did not ejaculate!* You have just had an orgasm without ejaculation.

What you want to do now is back off and rest a little bit by starting some really slow, easy thrusting. The slow, sensate-focus thrusting will help you maintain your erection. Give your partner lots of kisses for being so wonderful. But remember, it's not over yet. One down, one to go.

TROUBLESHOOTING TIP: After your first orgasm, your erection may go down temporarily. On a hardness scale of one to ten, it could drop as low as five. That is why you need to resume thrusting as soon as possible to bring yourself back "up" to speed.

Once you're both rested and ready, it's time to head for the home stretch. Start by intensifying your thrusting. Let your arousal level rise. But this time, *don't try to stop*. Pass Level 8. Keep thrusting. Pass Level 9. Keep thrusting. Thrust all the way through your point of no return. Pass GO. Collect $200. Let yourself have a full, fabulous orgasm, complete with ejaculation and eighty-piece orchestra accompaniment. *Congratulations! You have just had a multiple orgasm.* And boy, do you deserve it.

This exercise is called "The Big Takeoff" because it reminds me of the way airplanes take off at John Wayne International Airport in Orange County, California. To cut noise pollution on takeoff, the pilot angles the plane up really high, accelerates really fast, then cuts the engines. Your final peak at Level 9.9 should feel the same way. Your penis is angled up as high as it can go, you are thrusting as fast as you can, then suddenly you use your PC muscle to "cut the engines." Get the picture?

There is another image that helps my clients learn and remember this exercise. When you are doing this exercise, think of yourself running up a hill as fast as you can until you reach a sign that says "Level 8." You hit the brakes and catch your breath.

Maybe you slide back down the hill a little bit to the sign that says "Level 7." When you reach that sign, you start sprinting again. This time, you sprint all the way to the sign that says "Level 8.5" You hit the brakes again, catch your breath, and slide back down one level. These sprints continue to Level 9 and Level 9.5. Your last sprint is to the sign that says "Level 9.9: NO TRESPASSING BEYOND THIS POINT." Now this sign is just inches from the top of the hill, and beyond that is a steep drop to the bottom. So this time, you sprint as fast as you can up to the sign and hit your breaks really hard because you don't want to go over that hill. But even though your feet are firmly planted at the sign, your emotional momentum still makes you feel as though you've gone over the top, and you experience all the sensations of falling without actually falling.

These two images—the noise abatement takeoff and hillside sprints—should help you get your motion and your angles right at the crucial points in this exercise. If you already have an image of your own, use it by all means. I just find these two particular images extremely helpful when someone is learning these techniques for the first time. Some clients tell me that years after they have learned these techniques they still get a little misty eyed every time they fly out of John Wayne International Airport.

For the Do-It-Yourselfer

Some day, there will be an old saying, "You don't have to have a partner to have a multiple orgasm." Today, you just have to take my word for it. The following method is the one I use most often to teach

men how to have a multiple orgasm without a partner. Even if you have a partner to learn with, practicing on your own always accelerates the learning
process. This is a particularly good exercise to practice various techniques and hone your control. Most
men wind up slipping in at least a few private practice sessions when they are first learning these
methods. There's a lot to learn in the beginning, and
men tell me that practicing on their own helps build
their confidence.

Exercise 18: Two-Time Champion (solo)

Lie down and get very comfortable, or sit in a comfortable chair. Take some lubrication and begin
stroking your penis with a sensate focus genital
caress. We're going to start by doing some nice,
slow low-level peaks. I recommend doing one or
two Level 4 peaks, followed by a Level 5 peak and a
Level 6 peak. Each peak should last at least three or
four minutes.

Once you have completed at least three or four
low-level peaks, you're going to target Level 8. But
this time, you're going to do something a little bit
different.

TROUBLESHOOTING TIP: This technique
does not work if you try to jump into the
deep end of the pool and start with high-
level peaks like Level 8 or Level 9. You must
start slowly, practicing peaks at Level 4,
Level 5, and Level 6.

Instead of using a slow sensate focus stroke, you are going to stroke your penis as fast as you can to bring your arousal to Level 8.

When you reach Level 8, slam on your PC muscle, take a deep breath—as deep as you can—and open your eyes. Slow your stroking down and let your arousal drop a couple of levels.

Your next target is going to be Level 8.5. To get there, start stroking your penis as fast as you can. When you reach Level 8.5, squeeze your PC muscle as hard as you can, take a deep, deep breath, and open your eyes. Slow down your stroke, breathe really slow, and let your arousal drop again.

You're going to repeat this quick-stroke method for Level 9 and Level 9.5. Once you've completed these two levels, you're ready to stroke yourself as fast as you can all the way up to your point of inevitability—Level 9.9. When you hit that point, you want to squeeze that PC muscle as hard as you possibly can. Open your eyes. Breathe deeply. Hold that squeeze tight for at least a full five seconds, if not more.

At this point, your body should go into orgasm, but if your PC muscle is strong and you timed your squeeze right, you will not ejaculate.

This is hard work. You're probably sweating and gasping for breath right now if you've been following my instructions carefully. So let yourself drop a couple of levels and really catch your breath. Don't stop stroking because you don't want to lose your erection. Just stroke yourself slowly for a little while.

Ready for your second orgasm? Great. Once again, begin stroking your penis as fast as you can.

Pass Level 9, pass Level 9.5, and keep stroking. Stroke all the way through your point of inevitability into orgasm. Don't try to stop. Don't use your PC brake. Just let yourself have a full orgasm, complete with ejaculation. And that is how to have a beautiful do-it-yourself multiple orgasm. Now hit the showers.

You Know It's Working When . . .

Let me remind you one last time that your initial attempts with these multiple-orgasm exercises might bring strange or unusual results. You may only have a partial orgasm that doesn't feel all that special, or you may feel as though you missed an orgasm. You may even have a partial ejaculation without any orgasm after your first orgasm. Don't get scared and don't get discouraged. This is all very good news. You are clearly on your way to having your first full multiple orgasm. Your body is just getting adjusted to some new ideas. As I said before, most men have at least one of these unusual experiences before their techniques "click." So just relax and enjoy the process.

CHAPTER ELEVEN

Practice, Practice, Practice

Learning the techniques in this book is like learning anything new. Some guys will be just plain lucky. They will become multiorgasmic quickly and easily, and retain that ability, even improve upon it, for the rest of their lives. But what about everyone else? It's my experience that most men master the art of multiple orgasm in a more conventional two steps forward, one step backward fashion. For these men, the key to improvement is that one word we all dread: *practice*.

Don't you just hate it when a teacher starts lecturing you about the importance of practice? I know I do. That's why I stopped taking violin lessons four times. But . . . sigh . . . as we all know, sometimes there's just no substitute for putting the old nose to the grindstone.

You are learning to do amazing things with your body. It's not fair to expect yourself to be perfect the first time and every time. With a little bit of the "p" word, however, you can easily solidify and refine the techniques that will give you years and years of multiple pleasures. The most important thing to remember is that following these techniques will always bring results. Besides, there are worse things to be practicing on a Saturday night.

One easy way to strenghten your technique is to keep repeating the exercises you've just completed in chapter 10. Now I don't know about you, but that doesn't sound like a very painful homework assignment to me . . . and I hate homework. It is also very helpful to return to the exercises in earlier chapters that stress control and technique. Practice peaking (Exercises 6 and 7), peaking with the PC (Exercises 8, 9, and 10), and plateauing (Exercises 11 and 12).

These are especially helpful if you have a little trouble controlling your high-level peaks. Of course, you should *always* be giving your PC a workout to keep that wonderful little muscle strong as a vise.

There is one other exercise that really focuses on fine-tuning your timing and control. It's a really exciting exercise, and even if you don't try it, you should read through it. You may pick up an idea or two for later.

Exercise 19: Splitting the Atom (with a partner)

This exercise begins with the man lying on his back while his partner gives him a genital caress. Start by doing some really easy, low-level peaks or plateaus, say Level 4, Level 5, and Level 6. Take your time—at least four or five minutes at each level. Focus on the sensations of the caress.

Assuming that you have a good erection at this point, it's time to switch positions. Your partner should lie on her back with her legs up and knees bent. As you enter your partner, be certain that your weight is being supported by your legs, not your arms. Start thrusting at a medium pace.

Try to peak at Level 8. When you reach Level 8, slow down a bit and give your PC muscle a squeeze. Make it a medium squeeze, not a crusher. Your partner should slow down her movements to match yours. Let your arousal drop a level. Now pick up your speed and peak to Level 8.5. Slow down once again and give your PC another medium squeeze. Once again, your partner should slow down her movements to match yours. Let your arousal drop a level. Pick up your speed again and peak to Level 9. Slow down. Squeeze your PC and let your level drop. Each of these peaks should last at least three or four minutes.

Now this is where it gets a little bit more interesting than usual. From this point forward, you're going to be inching your way toward the point of inevitability, doing a series of short peaks (forty-five seconds or less) at higher and higher levels. Think of yourself as trying to do a peak at Level 9.1, Level 9.2, Level 9.3, etc., all the way up to Level 9.9.

It may sound a bit ridiculous to try and split hairs like this, but actually, it isn't that hard. For example, the difference between Level 9.4 and Level 9.5 is probably just a few thrusts—it could even be a single thrust. So what you're going to be doing is adding no more than a few additional thrusts every time you peak, using your PC muscle to bring you back down a bit in between each peak.

Your final peak will be at your point of inevitability—Level 9.9. Because of the gradual approach you have made to reach the top, you will probably find it much easier to squeeze your PC muscle at just the right moment this time, letting your body go over into orgasm without ejaculating.

After your first orgasm, give yourself a short rest by doing some very slow thrusting and some real easy breathing. Are you ready for more? If you're maintaining your erection and your arousal is pretty high, pick up your speed and thrust all the way through your point of inevitability, having a second orgasm, complete with ejaculation.

This exercise is very unusual for both partners because it's almost as if you're doing a very high-level plateau while squeezing your PC muscle every few seconds. It might feel as though your body is having little spasms or mini-orgasms before you have your first big orgasm.

If you miss one of your high-level peaks and wind up having a partial ejaculation, or even a full ejaculation with your first orgasm, that's perfectly okay. This is a pleasure technique, not a birth control technique, and there are no grades here. Try to have another peak and another orgasm, but if you can't recover, don't sweat it. Just remember that the next time you do this exercise, you're going to try to be a little bit more conservative with your thrusting.

Like most of the techniques you have now learned, this practice exercise can also be done without a partner. In fact, it's a particularly good exercise to do by yourself because it is a little bit easier to control the intensity of stimulation to the penis when you are using your own hands. Since we're working with such subtle incremental changes here, every little bit of control makes a difference.

Exercise 20: The Daily Double (solo)

The first thing you need to do is lie down and get comfortable, or sit in a very comfortable chair. Using plenty of lubrication, begin a sensate focus genital caress, slowly stroking your penis in a way that pleases you most. For the first part of this exercise, I'd just like you to do three or four low-level peaks (e.g., Level 4, Level 5, and Level 6), using your PC muscle to control your arousal at each peak. Try to use a medium-strength squeeze here, not a bone-crushing monster squeeze. Remember to breathe deeply at each peak to help bring your arousal back down a notch or two. Take your time. Each peak should take at least three or four minutes.

Your next peak is going to be a slightly more intense, Level 8 peak. You're probably stroking your penis a bit faster by now. That's fine, as long as you're not trying to rush the process. Keep using that PC muscle to control your arousal (a firm squeeze, but not a killer), and remember to breathe deeply as you squeeze. The next phase of this practice exercise begins at Level 9. Try to create a series of mini-peaks at Level 9, Level 9.1, Level 9.2, Level 9.3, etc., all the way to Level 9.9.

This sounds tricky, but it's not that hard once you know that it only takes two or three extra strokes to raise you from one mini-level to the next. So, let's say you've just used your PC muscle to peak at Level 9. Resume your caress and go three or four strokes past Level 9—this is Level 9.1. At Level 9.1, give your PC a medium squeeze, breathe deeply, and let your level drop ever so slightly (not even one full level). Start stroking yourself again. This time, go three or four strokes past Level 9.1— this is Level 9.2. Give your PC a medium squeeze and breathe deeply, letting your level drop again. Resume your caress. You are going to try to continue in this fashion, one tiny increment at a time, until you have worked yourself all the way up to Level 9.9.

By the time you reach Level 9.9, you should find it relatively easy to give that PC muscle one last solid squeeze at just the right moment, enabling your body to go into orgasm without having an ejaculation. As I stressed in the previous exercise, there is no need to fret if you miss one or two of these mini-levels and find yourself having a partial or full ejaculation. Just make a note to be more conservative with your stroking the next time you decide to practice (i.e., fewer strokes and/or slower strokes).

After your first orgasm, let yourself relax for a minute or two by doing some slow, even stroking. If you're still in the mood for more (this exercise is pretty exhausting and you may have had enough for one session), pick up your speed again and stroke yourself all the way to a second orgasm. This time, don't try to hold back your ejaculation.

Where Do You Go from Here?

How are you feeling right now? Having your first multiple orgasm can be a life-altering experience. It's disorienting to realize the effect this process will have on everything from your deepest fears to your deepest fantasies. One of the most rewarding moments for me as a clinician is when a client "gets it" for the first time. To be present for that moment when a person's understanding of his own sexual potential changes forever is quite a privilege. Obviously, I can't be with each and every one of you right now. But believe me that I am with you in spirit, and that I am truly proud of the work each of you has done.

Once you have taken control of the process you have just learned, multiple orgasms are easy. At first, you'll probably want to stick closely to the style and steps of the exercises. But before long, you're going to feel so confident in your ejaculatory control that you will be ready to expand your horizons. For the ambitious man and his partner, a brave new world awaits. Think of all the exercises in this book as your "starter kit." I've included everything you need to get going, and have hours and hours of fun, but it's really just the beginning. Soon you're going to want to accessorize.

I'm sure you have noticed by now that in each of the multiple-orgasm exercises in this book, I encouraged you to have your second orgasm within a minute or two of your first. The reason for suggesting you have your second orgasm so quickly was to make learning these techniques less overwhelming. It's hard enough to get to the point where you can have your first nonejaculatory orgasm. You don't need to be worrying about your second orgasm too. In the beginning, it's more important to know that you *can* have a second orgasm. The timing of that orgasm is a lot less important.

But now you know you can have two orgasms in a row without losing your erection. Now you're a believer. You may not want to have that second orgasm so quickly. No . . . you may want to wait a while . . . and wait . . . and wait. After all, isn't that what you're here for?

It's time to start expanding your repertoire. Most exercise regimens begin with stretching exercises, but that's where ours is going to end. Begin by trying to stretch out the time between your first and second orgasm. How long can you go before having your second orgasm? How long do you *want* to go?

Maybe you don't want to ejaculate the second time either, so you can have a third orgasm . . . or even a fourth orgasm! Why not? You've earned it. From now on, here is your new mantra: Stretch, stretch, stretch. Start experimenting too. Be creative and be ambitious. Now that you know what to do, you're in control. Just keep in mind that you always have your tried and true starter kit exercises to fall back on should you lose your way. Experiment with your timing. Experiment with your techniques, with your pacing, and with your positions. But before you do anything, *get your partner's input*. What does she want right now? What are her fantasies? What are her needs? Where does she want to go from here? Let her answers be your guide.

Male multiple orgasm is a magical thing. Magical for you, magical for your partner, and magical for the relationship. The hardest work is now behind you, and the future is full of possibilities. Just remember that wherever you decide to go from here, the most important thing for both of you is to *enjoy yourselves*.

CHAPTER TWELVE

Success!

I would like to end this book by introducing you to four more multiorgasmic men. All of these men have recently learned the very same techniques you are now practicing. Each man has a slightly different story to tell, and every story is well worth telling. While each of these men started with a different motivation, a different understanding of male sexuality, a different attitude, and a different physiology, they all had the same goal: male multiple orgasm. Having now achieved that goal, they all were eager to share their experiences with you, the reader. Some of them even had advice they wanted to offer.

Stephen's Story

Like many men who are interested in learning how to become multiorgasmic, Stephen's motivation was a natural outgrowth of his pleasure orientation. When we first met, he gave me the following information about himself:

"I believe there is so much pleasure to get out of every single aspect of life. No matter what it is I'm doing—skiing, biking, painting, even working—I'm always trying to find the pleasure zone and stretch my experience in that zone. To me, that's what life is all about. Of course, I've always tried to do the same thing with sex. I'm always experimenting with different techniques, always trying to expand 'the zone.' Don't get me wrong—it's not an obsession or anything like that. I just have a very strong internal drive, coupled with unending curiosity and a willingness to try new things.

"That's why I was so drawn to the idea of male multiple orgasm. The whole concept felt like such a natural extension of my attitude and my life. I still remember my reaction the first time I heard that such a thing existed. I was listening to some sexologist on the radio talking about the original Kinsey findings. It was a pretty boring discussion, until he mentioned the part about multiorgasmic men. Suddenly, a big smile broke across my face, and I said to my girlfriend, 'Now that sounds like it should be me.'"

Stephen's goal when he started working with me at the clinic was to learn how he could stay inside his partner's vagina at very high arousal levels for as long as possible. He told me that he didn't want "just any old multiple orgasm." He was looking for an experience of maximum intensity. That really made me laugh, since I tend to think of almost every multiple orgasm as a pretty intense experience.

This is how Stephen summed up his learning process:

"After mastering the initial exercises, it wasn't long before I learned how to maintain my erection and my arousal after my first orgasm. At first, I wasn't always able to stop myself from ejaculating. This didn't surprise me. After all, I've been ejaculating during orgasm for a lot of years and my body has to be pretty used to that path. . . . I didn't expect to get total control overnight.

"Even if I ejaculated I would try to continue thrusting for as long as possible. Dina, my partner, was extremely helpful during those times. She never judged me, never criticized me, and most important, never tried to stop me. She just let me do whatever I could do. I was determined to get the hang of this one way or the other, but her generous attitude really helped.

"Soon I was able to have a second orgasm within two or three minutes of my first. But that was just the beginning. Once I knew I could keep my erection and keep going, I really started to push 'the zone.' Five minutes, ten minutes, fifteen, twenty. . . . I find that now I can even let myself ejaculate during my first orgasm without losing my erection, and I still have a second, partial ejaculation with my second orgasm. That, to me, is amazing.

"The key, I have discovered, has been to focus everything on the sensation of moving in and out of my partner's body. That's where the sensate focus exercises really paid off. When Dina is wet from my first ejaculation, the experience is even more intense. I guess that's what helps make the 'impossible' now possible."

Alex's Story

When Alex was a teenager, he was able to have multiple orgasms with many of the women with whom he was having sex. He was very self-assured, and really loved having sex. As he got older, however, he lost his multiorgasmic ability. He also lost a lot of his sexual confidence.

Alex came to my office with his wife Paula. They had been married for six years. While they assured me that many aspects of their sex life were very rewarding, they also acknowledged that there were areas that needed work.

During this first visit, Alex expressed a very powerful desire to enhance and control his sexual response, and to recapture the magic of his teenage years. Paula's greatest concern was Alex's lack of confidence, but she was also intrigued by the idea of male multiple orgasm, and had no trouble imagining the possible benefits for both of them.

Alex started his relearning process by strengthening his PC muscle. He then began doing peaking and plateauing exercises with Paula during intercourse. Here is how he recalled his initial sessions with Paula practicing these new techniques:

"During intercourse with Paula I would squeeze my PC at each peak, all the way up to the point of inevitability. At that point, I would have what I would call a '60-percent orgasm' along with a partial ejaculation. I was able to maintain my erection, and continue having intercourse with Paula, which was good. But frankly, it didn't *feel* that good. It actually felt kind of funny—weird funny—and at that point I was skeptical."

After talking to Alex and Paula about these initial experiences, I realized that Alex had not been highly successful his first few times. I felt that Alex needed to back up a bit and slow his process down. Instead of pushing him to keep practicing the techniques he was already using, I encouraged him to do more awareness exercises.

As a couple, I thought Alex and Paula would benefit from more practice doing sensate focus caresses. And I suspected that Alex would also benefit from focusing more on the process of creating and maintaining plateaus at higher and higher levels. I suggested he practice his plateaus alone at first to keep some of the pressure off. That helped a lot, as Alex illustrates:

"I started to practice by myself, doing plateaus at Level 8, 8.5, 9, and 9.5. At the point of inevitability I would focus intently on my groin and the sensation of thrusting. At this point, I had a sense of an extremely prolonged orgasm—maybe ten to twelve seconds, compared to my usual three to four seconds. I would be sweating like they do in the movies and my heart would be pounding. That was a very new experience for me, and it was very intense. I remember that at the time I was thinking to myself, 'You may be on to something here.'

"Then I tried doing the squeeze again during intercourse with Paula. The first three times I tried, I only had a '50-percent orgasm,' but unlike the previous times, I was no longer ejaculating. Something about my body was definitely changing, and I felt really encouraged."

At this point in the training process I decided it was time to introduce Alex and Paula to my favorite exercise: "The Big Takeoff." Alex recalls:

"Learning the new exercise was the final turning point for us. The *very first time* Paula and I tried this, I had two '100-percent orgasms' within seven minutes of each other. Paula also had an extraordinary orgasm. Success!

"At first, it was easier to have my second orgasm outside of Paula's vagina. Once she felt satisfied, we would stop having intercourse and she would masturbate me to my climax with her hands. That was fine for a while, but eventually I became comfortable staying inside her for my second climax. Of course, that felt better for her *and* for me.

"I cannot overstate what becoming multiorgasmic again has done for me. Within less than two months I went from being extremely uncertain about the whole thing to being able to have two '100-percent orgasms'—one without an ejaculation and one with—whenever I chose to do so. Becoming multiorgasmic has given me back my sexual confidence, and a sense of myself that is hard to put in words. Paula teases me about it all the time. She says that I'm a different person—a person she wants to have sex with a lot more often."

Charles's Story

Charles competes every year in a number of marathons and biathlons. Being a serious athlete, he was prepared to build up his techniques the same way an athlete would build up endurance for a marathon or other sporting event. Charles knew his body well enough to know that if he was patient, he could train himself to have a multiorgasmic response almost automatically. Here's what he had to say:

"I love sex, and my wife and I have great fun together in bed, but there is a part of me that takes sex very seriously. I have pushed my body hard through all kinds of rigorous athletic training programs, and it has always paid off in the end. Intuitively, I knew that it wouldn't be any different for something like male multiple orgasm. You put yourself through your paces, you get the result.

"My strategy was to do an exercise and learn a technique by myself, then try the same technique in a session with my wife. The sessions with my wife were strictly for our pleasure. I did the hard work by myself."

Charles was anxious to get started, yet he progressed through his training slowly and methodically—the mark of an athlete who takes his work seriously. He explains:

"I exercised my PC muscle a lot, but I never overdid it; I knew it would only be a matter of time before everything kicked in. People push too hard when they don't know their bodies. But serious athletes have learned the rewards of pacing themselves. Why should it be any different with these exercises?"

Did Charles's patience and hard work pay off? I'll let him tell you:

"It has been almost a year now since I started to learn these techniques, and the results have been extraordinary. Compared to other exercise regimens of mine, this one was a snap. I never needed to learn the 'windsprint' technique. All I had to do was practice my peaking, plateauing, and PC control and everything else unfolded effortlessly. I couldn't really tell you why I didn't need the final exercises. My body just found a different way."

There are many paths to the top of the mountain, and clearly, Charles found his. The goal here is male multiple orgasm, and as far as I'm concerned, whatever works, works. Not surprisingly, it's still working for Charles:

"When a marathon is over, it's over, but when you're multiorgasmic, it never ends. I am becoming more and more orgasmic all the time, even though I don't even try anymore. I have had as many as five orgasms during one session of intercourse with my wife. You know what the odd part is? It's as though I've suddenly discovered that my body is naturally multiorgasmic. I never knew it because I didn't even know that such a thing existed. But now it feels like it's who I am, and who I always was.

"My wife says that knowing me and knowing how determined I can be, she's not entirely surprised by my success, though she certainly is pleased. She thinks this all happened so easily for me because I'm so driven, but I think that's only half of the story. I really wonder how many men are probably just like me, with this 'natural' ability just sitting there, waiting to be tapped."

Frederick's Story

Finally, I'd like you to meet Frederick. Frederick is a structural engineer who told me that his desire to learn about male multiple orgasm was driven by "an engineer's fascination with how his body works." Men like Frederick are so methodical and scientific in their style of approach that from the very beginning their success seems inevitable.

To train his body to respond the way he envisioned it could, Frederick invented his own style of "riding the 9's." He learned to plateau at Level 9 for a full ten minutes, using a combination of breathing, PC contractions, and varying the speed of his thrusting. You learned to create plateaus like this in chapter 7, but you probably didn't imagine you could ride high-level plateaus all the way to orgasm. Well, Frederick did, and he liked the results so much that he stuck with it, creating his own personal style of climaxing.

Riding a wave like this at very high levels is different from the more aggressive techniques you learned in chapter 10. Instead of pushing yourself to the point of orgasm, you almost fall over into orgasm after plateauing for long intervals at very high levels. As I briefly mentioned earlier in the book, this type of approach most closely resembles the way many women have multiple orgasms.

Not surprisingly, Frederick had a lot to say about his process:

"I did most of my training by myself. I was able to bring myself to multiple orgasm before I tried doing it with a partner. If I can be frank here, I've always felt that masturbation is essential if you're going to learn your own personal response. I know that some people might be uncomfortable with this, but personally, I think they are getting in the way of their own progress and their own pleasure.

"If you're like me, the kind of guy who can get pretty obsessed with mastering something like this, I don't think it's fair to ask your partner to work with you every single time you want to practice these techniques. Sometimes? Yes. But not every single time. Still, that practice is important—at least it was for me. I couldn't imagine learning to have the kind of control I now have if I didn't spend a lot of time working on this alone."

Frederick has learned to have as many as *four* orgasms before he ejaculates. His final words on the subject should be an inspiration to every man:

"You can't fail! If you do the work, you simply cannot fail! Every exercise is a stepping stone closer to the goal. Each one, no matter how it feels, is a learning experience. Sometimes it works, sometimes it doesn't, and sometimes you don't know whether it did or it didn't. That can be a little weird, but your body keeps changing; it keeps adjusting and adapting. The most important thing is to keep a positive attitude all the time and just keep going. And keep working that PC muscle! A strong PC muscle is a requirement for success!"

Your Story

So there you have it. Four very different men, four very different experiences, yet every one is a success story.

So what about you? What's your story? I want to know. Why did you decide to learn about male multiple orgasm? What has the learning experience been like for you? What was easy? What was challenging? Now that you have completed all of the exercises, what does it feel like to be a multiorgasmic man? How has your body changed? How has your sense of yourself changed? If you are in a relationship, how has that changed? What has been your partner's experience of this process? What advice do you have for other men who are interested in learning these techniques? I'm really interested in your input. Let me know by writing to me care of the publisher.

Interesting Things to Read When You're Not Having Sex

Anand, M. (1989). *The Art of Sexual Ecstasy*. Los Angeles, CA: Jeremy P. Tarcher, Inc. Interesting "ecstasy" exercises for men, women, and couples.

Barbach, L. (1975). *For Yourself: The Fulfillment of Female Sexuality*. New York: Doubleday and Company. For the ladies, and the men who love them, this book focuses on increased orgasmic response for women.

Brauer, A., and Brauer, D. (1983). *ESO* (extended sexual orgasm). New York: Warner Books. Packed with orgasm-enhancement exercises for men and women. Interesting to read and fun to try.

Carter, S., and Sokol, J. (1988). *What Really Happens in Bed*. New York: Evans. A solid, sane look at sexual fears, sexual fantasies, and sexual realities. Smart, smart, smart.

Danoff, D. (1993). *Superpotency*. New York: Warner Books. Helpful for men who are trying to develop a more positive attitude about their sexuality.

Dunn, M., and Trost, J. (1989). Male multiple orgasms: A descriptive study. *Archives of Sexual Behavior* 18(5), 377–387. One of the more important journal articles concerning the existence of male multiple orgasm and non-ejaculatory orgasm. A must-read for any doubting Thomas.

Eichel, E., and Nobile, P. (1991). *The Perfect Fit: How to Achieve Mutual Fulfillment and Monogamous Passion Through the New Intercourse*. New York: Donald I. Fine. The title says it all.

Hartman, W., and Fithian, M. (1984). *Any Man Can*. New York: St. Martin's Press. One of the first books to discuss male multiple orgasm in depth and offer possible means of achieving it.

Keesling, B. (1993). *Sexual Pleasure*. Alameda, CA: Hunter House. One of my personal favorites (surprise, surprise). If you're having real trouble with your ejaculatory control, check out the exercises in this book. There's lots in here for women as well.

Kennedy, A., and Dean, S. (1986). *Touching for Pleasure—A Guide to Sensual Enhancement*. Chatsworth, CA: Chatsworth Press. A book that focuses on touching—I think that's important.

Kinsey, A., Pomeroy, W., and Martin, C. (1948). *Sexual Behavior in the Human Male*. Philadelphia: W. B. Saunders Company. The classic study that redefined our understanding of male sexuality. A must for every library.

Ladas, A., Whipple, B., and Perry, J. (1982). *The G Spot and Other Recent Discoveries About Human Sexuality*. New York: Dell Publishing Co., Inc. Still controversial after over a decade—the debate rages on.

Montagu, A. (1986, 3rd edition). *Touching: The Human Significance of the Skin*. New York: Harper & Row. Sensitive, sensuous, and helpful reading.

Penney, A. (1993). *How to Make Love to a Man (Safely)*. New York: Carol Southern Books. An easy, smart read that has something for women *and* men. It's the nineties, and sex is no good unless it's safe.

Ramsdale, D., and Ramsdale, E. (1990, 9th printing). *Sexual Energy Ecstasy: A Practical Guide to Lovemaking Secrets of the East and West*. Playa del Rey, CA: Peak Skill Publishing. Very advanced ideas and techniques for the curious and the motivated.

Robbins, M., and Jensey, G. (1978). Multiple orgasm in males. *The Journal of Sex Research* 14(1), 21–26. One of the earliest studies suggesting that men could *learn* to have nonejaculatory orgasms and multiple orgasms. Check it out.

Schwartz, B. (1989). *The One Hour Orgasm*. Houston, TX: Breakthru Publishing. Why rush a good thing? Valuable exercises are included.

Thornton, J. (1992). Multiple orgasm. *Self*, May 1992, pp. 158–161. An important magazine piece for those who don't like struggling through professional journals.

Zilbergeld, B. (1992). *The New Male Sexuality*. New York: Bantam Books. Another classic that helps take men out of the sexual dark ages.

Male Sexual Organs

urinary bladder

prostate gland

urethral bulb (swollen
at end of emission
phase)

vas deferens

penis

urethra

PC muscle

testicle

Male sexuality anatomy—relevant to ejaculation.
I have left out several major organs in order to
simplify the ejaculatory system.